House Officer
S E R I E S

Urology

Fourth Edition

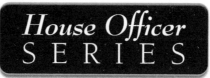

House Officer
S E R I E S

Urology

Fourth Edition

Michael T. Macfarlane, M.D.
Louisville, Kentucky

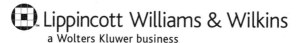

Lippincott Williams & Wilkins
a Wolters Kluwer business

Philadelphia · Baltimore · New York · London
Buenos Aires · Hong Kong · Sydney · Tokyo

Acquisitions Editor: Brian Brown
Developmental Editor: Maria McAvey
Project Manager: Jennifer Harper
Senior Manufacturing Manager: Benjamin Rivera
Marketing Manager: Adam Glazer
Creative Director: Doug Smock
Production Services: Nesbitt Graphics, Inc.
Printer: R.R. Donnelley, Crawfordsville

© 2006 by LIPPINCOTT WILLIAMS & WILKINS, a Wolters Kluwer business
530 Walnut Street
Philadelphia, PA 19106 USA
LWW.com

Third edition, © 2001 Lippincott Williams & Wilkins
Second edition, © 1995 Williams & Wilkins
First edition, © 1988 Williams & Wilkins

Printed in the USA

Library of Congress Cataloging-in-Publication Data
Macfarlane, Michael T.
   Urology/Michael T. Macfarlane.—4th ed.
      p. ; cm.—(House officer series)
   Includes bibliographical references and index.
   ISBN 0-7817-9933-3 (alk. paper)
   1. Urology—Handbooks, manuals, etc.   2. Genitourinary organs—
Diseases—Handbooks, manuals, etc.   I. Title.   II. Series.
   [DNLM: 1. Urologic Diseases—Handbooks.   WJ 39 M1435ua 2006]
RC872.9.M33 2006
616.6—dc22
                                                                            2006007347

Care has been taken to confirm the accuracy of the information presented and to describe generally accepted practices. However, the author and publisher are not responsible for errors or omissions or for any consequences from application of the information in this book and make no warranty, expressed or implied, with respect to the currency, completeness, or accuracy of the contents of the publication. Application of this information in a particular situation remains the professional responsibility of the practitioner.

The author and publisher have exerted every effort to ensure that drug selection and dosage set forth in this text are in accordance with current recommendations and practice at the time of publication. However, in view of ongoing research, changes in government regulations, and the constant flow of information relating to drug therapy and drug reactions, the reader is urged to check the package insert for each drug for any change in indications and dosage and for added warnings and precautions. This is particularly important when the recommended agent is a new or infrequently employed drug.

Some drugs and medical devices presented in this publication have Food and Drug Administration (FDA) clearance for limited use in restricted research settings. It is the responsibility of the health care provider to ascertain the FDA status of each drug or device planned for use in their clinical practice.

To purchase additional copies of this book, call our customer service department at (800) 638-3030 or fax orders to (301) 223-2320. International customers should call (301) 223-2300.

Visit Lippincott Williams & Wilkins on the Internet: at LWW.com. Lippincott Williams & Wilkins customer service representatives are available from 8:30 am to 6pm, EST.

10 9 8 7 6 5 4 3 2

About the Author

Michael T. Macfarlane, M.D., graduated Alpha Omega Alpha (AOA) from the College of Physicians and Surgeons, Columbia University, New York, New York. After completing two years of general surgery training at the Brigham and Women's Hospital and Harvard Medical School in Boston, he went on to serve as resident in Urology at the UCLA School of Medicine in Los Angeles. While serving as Chief Resident at UCLA, he wrote the first edition of *Urology* for the House Officer. After completing his urologic residency, he stayed on as Assistant Professor of Surgery/Urology at UCLA and was the Chief of Urology at the Veterans Administration Medical Center, Sepulveda, California. Dr. Macfarlane is at present in the practice of urology and a Clinical Associate Professor of Surgery/Urology at the University of Louisville School of Medicine, Louisville, Kentucky.

Foreword to the First Edition (1988)

The field of urology has expanded rapidly during the past decade, and as new findings in the laboratory and in clinical research are brought into the realm of standard practice, the body of information promises to increase even more rapidly. Faced with this deluge of information, the new urology house officer must find innovative methods to evaluate and manage the spectrum of urologic problems with which he or she is faced on a daily basis. The enormous daily work load of the house officer precludes extensive daily library searches or reading sessions, and too often only a small portion of available knowledge is brought to bear on the multitude of clinical urology problems. Though a plethora of texts and journals has emerged in recent years, none effectively addresses the issue of quick reference for the novice in urology. Herein lies the great strength of this publication.

This book is divided into two major sections, Chief Presentations and Selected Topics. In the first section, almost every possible clinical situation that can be encountered by the house officer is outlined. This provides a quick reference to guide the physician in evaluating the patient and scheduling the necessary clinical and laboratory tests. The section on Selected Topics is an in-depth but brief discussion of urologic diseases, including their management. Useful tests and drugs along with the appropriate dosages and their potential toxicities are included. The discussions on management, unencumbered by lengthy referencing and detailed discussion of current debates and controversies, provide a balanced final analysis of the state of the art. The test is directed toward the more junior urology house officers but is well suited to medical students at all levels during their clinical rotations in urology. Indeed, physicians in other specialties, especially Family Practice and Internal Medicine, will undoubtedly be rewarded by this text, out of proportion to the small amount of time needed to extract the ready information required to manage their patients. The author is an energetic and talented urology house officer, who understands what students and junior house officers need to know. I am sure that *Urology* for the House Officer will become the gold standard of a whole genre of such publications.

Jean B. deKernion, M.D.

Professor of Surgery/Urology
Chief, Division of Urology
UCLA School of Medicine
Los Angeles, California

Preface to the Fourth Edition

The goal of this fourth edition of *Urology* (for the House Officer) is unchanged from that of the first, i.e., to create a concise source of clinical information on urology for medical students and residents that they can easily carry in their pockets and refer to quickly. The previous editions of this book were well received by both students and reviewers and have been translated into many languages. Since this book contains primarily the fundamentals of urology, much of it remains unchanged from previous editions. However, I have attempted to keep this book up to date with changes as they become accepted and established. Like other areas of medicine today, urologic practices are sometimes prematurely driven by corporate interests before adequate data are available to warrant their acceptance. I have tried to avoid introducing such information into a core text too early.

As with the previous editions, this manual primarily presents the nonsurgical aspects of urology— the information needed for making a diagnosis and deciding on the proper treatment course. This is a what-to-do book and not a how-to-do book. It does not include surgical technique or how to perform a particular procedure. Thus, it is also ideally suited to family practitioners and emergency room physicians who wish to quickly review a specific urologic presentation. It is not meant to be an all-encompassing treatise on urology. For more detailed reviews, refer to one of the standard urologic textbooks such *Campbell's Urology*. References have been omitted to keep the size and weight of the book small. A list of suggested readings is at the end of the text.

The format of the previous editions has been retained. The first part, Chief Presentations, covers the most common presenting complaints in the general urology clinic. It is intentionally handled in a cookbook-like fashion. Its goals are simple:

1. Define the problem.
2. State the differential diagnosis and outline the appropriate workup to make the correct diagnosis.
3. Begin therapeutic planning when applicable.

The second part, Selected Topics, covers the major areas of urology in greater detail. Again, it is not meant to substitute for reading the traditional textbooks. This part presents a concise review of these topics for quick study. When writing a short manual such as this, one is conflicted over writing too much or too little. This can occasionally result in oversimplification of otherwise complicated topics; however, brevity is necessary to accomplish the goals of this handbook.

> Michael T. Macfarlane, M.D.
> Clinical Associate Professor of Urology
> University of Louisville School of Medicine
> Louisville, Kentucky

Contents

Part One

Chief Presentations

1 Urinary Retention

Acute urinary retention is the sudden inability to void. It is a common problem that usually causes agonizing suprapubic pain that demands urgent relief.

ETIOLOGY

Acute urinary retention most commonly occurs in patients who have preexisting partial bladder outlet obstruction and experience a decrease in detrusor pressures or a sudden increase in outlet resistance. Frequent precipitating events include drugs (such as α-agonists, anticholinergics, antihistamines, and anesthetics), acute infection, bleeding, or overdistention of the bladder (e.g., that which happens after anesthesia).

Benign Prostatic Hyperplasia

Patients with increasing outlet resistance secondary to benign prostatic hyperplasia (BPH) may go into acute urinary retention by delaying voiding. With overdistention, the already weakened detrusor will become atonic. Edema from acute infection (e.g., prostatitis) can also send the patient into retention.

Stricture

An acute event such as infection, bleeding, or overdistention of the bladder can cause the patient with severe stricture disease to go into retention.

Blood Clots

Acute clot retention can occur secondary to bleeding from BPH or bladder tumor or be a late complication from transurethral resection of the prostate, particularly in patients on anticoagulants.

Sloughing of a scab within the prostatic fossa can produce significant bleeding with clot formation. Prostate needle biopsy can also be a precipitating event.

Bladder Neck Contracture

A tight scar formed at the bladder neck after transurethral resection of the prostate can lead to retention if infection, bleeding, or acute overdistention of the bladder occurs.

Prostate Cancer

Acute urinary retention can occur in patients with advanced cancer of the prostate. Patients will often give a history of rapid onset of obstructive voiding symptoms as opposed to the more gradual onset usually noted with BPH.

Myopathic Bladder

Detrusor myopathy can result from overdistention of the bladder. This is most frequently seen after surgery, when the normal voiding pattern is delayed while the patient recovers from anesthesia.

Neuropathic Bladder

An areflexic neurogenic bladder will be in retention if bladder outlet resistance is higher than intravesical pressures. These patients are usually managed on intermittent catheterization.

Medications

Anticholinergic agents, antihistamines, or α-agonists, all of which are common components of over-the-counter cold remedies, can cause retention in patients with mild to moderate prostatism.

Psychogenic Retention

Patients with psychogenic urinary retention have a persistent volitional override of detrusor contractility. This is not a surgical disease and should be treated with intermittent catheterization and psychiatric referral.

WORKUP

The workup for acute urinary retention is primarily directed at quickly determining the underlying urologic problem (e.g., stricture, BPH, prostate cancer).

History

Inquire about strictures, venereal disease, lower urinary tract symptoms, past urologic surgery (e.g., prostate surgery), and medications. Primary anticholinergic agents, drugs with anticholinergic side effects [e.g., diphenhydramine (Benadryl), antidepressants], or α-agonists [e.g., phenylephrine (Neo-Synephrine)] may precipitate urinary retention.

Physical Examination

Include a digital rectal examination (DRE) to assess the size of the prostate and careful palpation and percussion of the suprapubic area to confirm the presence of a full bladder.

MANAGEMENT

Initial management of the patient in retention is to provide urinary drainage by the least invasive technique available. Definitive treatment can be handled on an elective basis. It is generally recommended that more than 1,000 mL should not be drained from the bladder at once because of the possibility of a vasovagal reaction. After draining 1,000 mL, clamp the catheter for a few minutes before allowing the remainder to drain.

Lubrication

Liberal lubrication should always be used when attempting to pass any instrument into the urethra. Patients will often tightly contract their external sphincter muscles because of discomfort and anxiety. The use of 2% lidocaine (Xylocaine) jelly can make the difference between passing and not passing a catheter.

Foley Catheter

Simple placement of a Foley catheter is the treatment of choice; however, this occasionally can be a formidable task. Placement of a Foley in the patient with BPH can often be facilitated by using a large caliber (e.g., 22 F) catheter. The stiffness of the heavier catheter can help to separate the hypertrophied lateral lobes. Additionally, a prominent median lobe can be difficult to get over. The curve of a coudé tip catheter can be effective in negotiating the median lobe of the prostate. The coudé catheter is inserted with the curved tip pointing up toward the patient's head. A urethral stricture should be suspected if catheter passage is blocked in the distal or anterior urethra. Small catheters can often be used to pass a strictured area; sometimes a feeding tube as small as 8 F may be necessary.

Percutaneous Suprapubic Tube

Insertion of a percutaneous suprapubic tube requires that the bladder contain at least 200 to 300 mL; however, the fuller the better. The bladder should be easily percussed in the suprapubic region. If percussion is difficult, ultrasound can be used to confirm that the bladder is full. Previous lower abdominal surgery is a contraindication to attempting percutaneous placement because adhesions may hold a loop of bowel in the area of insertion. Other contraindications to percutaneous placement of a suprapubic tube are listed in the following section.

▓ Contraindications to Percutaneous Suprapubic Tube

- Previous lower abdominal surgery
- A small contracted neurogenic bladder
- Coagulopathy
- Known bladder tumor

Many different prepackaged suprapubic tube kits are available, such as the Stamey catheter. Percutaneous suprapubic tubes are generally ineffective for draining patients with clot retention because of their small caliber. Open surgical placement of a large caliber tube is necessary in this case if urethral catheterization is impossible.

Filiforms and Followers

Filiforms are long, thin, fiberglass probes with straight or spiral tips that are inserted into the urethra. With careful manipulation, they can often negotiate narrow strictures and pass into the bladder. Followers are tapered stiff catheters that screw into the end of the filiform and can follow the filiform through the stricture area into the bladder. By using progressively larger caliber followers, the stricture area can be dilated up to allow passage of a standard Foley catheter. The stricture should be dilated to 2 F greater than the catheter that will be inserted. An open-tipped catheter can be placed over a Councill stylet and follow the filiform into the bladder. The stylet and filiform can then be removed, leaving the catheter in place. Filiforms and followers should not be used for the first time without experienced supervision. They can cause serious injury to the urethra or rectum.

Cystourethroscopy

In difficult cases, the safest and most successful technique is to pass the filiform under direct vision using a cystoscope. A flexible cystoscope can be used in the office setting or brought to the patient's bedside in the hospital or emergency room. The filiform is passed alongside the cystoscope and visually guided through the stricture. The scope is then removed and the stricture dilated with followers. Cystoscopy is also beneficial in negotiating a posterior urethral false passage created by prior attempts to insert a catheter.

COMPLICATIONS OF RELIEVING OBSTRUCTION

Postobstructive Diuresis

Patients may require careful monitoring for postobstructive diuresis (>200 mL/hour) after establishing drainage, particularly if obstruction was prolonged and blood urea nitrogen (BUN) and creatinine are significantly elevated (see Chapter 29).

Hemorrhage

Relief of longstanding obstruction *may* result in major hematuria secondary to bladder mucosal disruption. These patients will need careful monitoring and continuous bladder irrigation. In severe cases, more rigorous measures may be necessary (see Chapter 4).

Hypotension

Significant hypotension may occur secondary to a vasovagal response or may be caused by relief of pelvic venous compression from bladder distention.

Lower Urinary Tract Symptoms

Lower urinary tract symptoms (LUTS) are classified as storage symptoms (previously referred to as irritative symptoms) or voiding symptoms (previously referred to as obstructive symptoms). This change in terminology, recommended by the World Health Organization, can be applied to any patient with urinary symptoms, regardless of age or sex.

STORAGE (IRRITATIVE) SYMPTOMS

Storage (irritative) symptoms (e.g., frequency, nocturia, urgency, incontinence, and bladder pain) are common presenting complaints that may herald several different urologic diseases. Storage symptoms tend to be the most bothersome to the patient, particularly nocturia.

Frequency describes the need to urinate more often than usual. If polyuria (large urine volume) is excluded, then the patient has a functionally reduced bladder capacity by virtue of decreased compliance, residual urine, or pain on stretching. Causes include infection, tumor, stone, outlet obstruction, neurogenic bladder, or foreign body. Frequency is best recorded in terms of how many hours between voiding.

Nocturia describes the act of awakening at night to urinate and has a pathophysiology similar to that of frequency. Ask how many times the patient awakes from sleep to urinate and how much he or she drinks before retiring. Nocturia one to two times per night is inconsequential if the patient drinks a few cups of coffee before bed.

Urgency describes the patient's sensation to urinate immediately if an "accident" is to be avoided. Urgency most often accompanies infection, bladder outlet obstruction (BOO), or neurogenic bladder.

Incontinence is the involuntary loss of urine and is the ultimate sign of storage failure. Incontinence is frequently associated with urgency, frequency, or nocturia and should be distinguished by the different types (see Chapter 5).

Pain with storage is generally located in the suprapubic area and is a result of bladder distention. It is distinguished from the more common pain with voiding referred to as dysuria, which is also a classic irritative symptom categorized as a voiding symptom [see "Voiding (Obstructive) Symptoms"].

VOIDING (OBSTRUCTIVE) SYMPTOMS

Voiding (obstructive) symptoms include hesitancy, straining to void, poor stream, intermittency, dysuria, feeling of incomplete emptying, and terminal or postmicturition dribbling. A poor, slow, or weak stream is the complaint most directly associated with BOO. Other complaints include decreased force of stream, hesitancy in voiding, or difficulty starting the stream. Patients also complain of decreased caliber or narrowing of the stream, which may be split or interrupted. These are all symptoms of increased outlet resistance to urine flow in the urethra or bladder neck. Voiding symptoms, except for dysuria, occur primarily in males. Prostatic enlargement is the most common cause; however, other causes include urethral stricture, bladder neck contracture, and cancer of the prostate or urethra.

Dysuria describes a burning or painful sensation on urination, which is usually felt in the urethra. It is most commonly a symptom of urinary tract infection (UTI).

DIFFERENTIAL DIAGNOSIS

Benign Prostatic Enlargement

Benign prostatic enlargement occurs primarily in elderly males with symptoms that usually progress gradually over a long period. Patients typically present with frequency, nocturia, and a slow, weak stream secondary to benign prostatic hyperplasia (BPH). Urinalysis is often negative, peak uroflow is reduced (<10 mL/second), and a high postvoid residual urine may be noted.

Urethral Stricture

Strictures of the urethra can occur at any age. They occur more frequently in males with a history of venereal disease, trauma, or prior instrumentation.

Infection

Infection is probably the most common cause of storage symptoms. The patient with frequency and urgency, and pyuria on urinalysis, has a UTI. Dysuria is also a common symptom of infection. History and physical examination usually provide the additional information to localize the infection (e.g., cystitis, prostatitis, urethritis).

Acute Prostatitis

Edema and swelling of the posterior urethra, which occur with acute prostatitis, can cause significant outlet obstruction. The symptoms usually improve after the infection is eradicated. In addition to the poor flow, the patient will complain of frequency, dysuria, and high fever.

Bladder Tumor

Remember that up to 30% of patients with bladder cancer will present with irritative symptoms without hematuria. This is most often due to carcinoma in situ or muscle invasive bladder cancer. Therefore, the presence of persistent irritative symptoms in an adult with negative urinalysis and culture is an indication for cystoscopy and cytologies.

Cancer of the Prostate

Prostate cancer is another disease of elderly males, with 75% of cases occurring between the ages of 60 and 85 years. Voiding symptoms often occur more rapidly than with BPH, and the digital rectal examination (DRE) will usually be positive.

Bladder Neck Contracture

In the adult, bladder neck contracture occurs as a late complication of prostate surgery. Scar formation eventually narrows the bladder neck, increasing resistance and producing recurrent symptoms of BOO.

Meatal Stenosis

Meatal stenosis is a narrowing of the urethral opening on the glans penis. It is usually a congenital anomaly and can cause significant outlet resistance in the newborn.

Posterior Urethral Valves

Posterior urethral valves are congenital membranelike structures located in the distal prostatic urethra; they are the most common cause of BOO in male children. Diagnosis is made on voiding cystourethrography (VCUG) and cystourethroscopy.

Other (Stone, Foreign Body, Prolapsing Ureterocele)

Any foreign body or stone in the urethra or bladder can potentially obstruct the outlet. Irritation from the stone or foreign body can cause frequency and urgency. Urinalysis will usually reveal hematuria and pyuria. The diagnosis is made at cystoscopy. Rarely, a prolapsing ureterocele has been known to obstruct the bladder neck.

Neurogenic Bladder

Frequency and urgency are common symptoms of neurogenic bladder dysfunction. Association with urge incontinence or recurrent UTIs may be noted. A urodynamic investigation is indicated after infection, tumor, and outlet obstruction have been ruled out.

Overactive Bladder

Overactive bladder (OAB) is a condition characterized by a sudden, uncomfortable need to urinate with or without urine leakage usually with daytime and nighttime frequency, whose etiology cannot be clearly identified. It is primarily a diagnosis of exclusion and is managed for the most part by behavioral therapy and antimuscarinic medications.

Neurogenic Detrusor-Sphincter Dyssynergia

An uncoordinated detrusor sphincter reflex can result in significant obstruction to urine flow. This reflex is seen almost exclusively with spinal cord injury. A urodynamic evaluation is needed to confirm diagnosis.

Polyuria

Uncontrolled diabetes mellitus or diabetes insipidus can present with frequency and nocturia. Patients will report voiding large volumes and polydipsia. Urinalysis may show sugar on the dipstick. Patients on diuretic therapy and psychogenic water drinkers can also present with frequency and nocturia. Occasionally, patients with new onset congestive heart failure will present with nocturia. With recumbency at night, intravascular volume will be augmented by return of lower extremity edema fluid.

Pneumaturia and Fecaluria

Pneumaturia refers to the passage of air on urination, whereas fecaluria is the passage of fecal material during voiding. The passage of air or fecal matter in the urine is most commonly the result of a fistulous communication between the intestines and urinary tract, usually at the bladder or urethra. The fistula is generally the result of gastrointestinal disease—most commonly diverticulitis, colon cancer, or Crohn's disease. Patients will present with irritative symptoms and UTI in addition to the complaints of pneumaturia and fecaluria. The diagnosis is confirmed by cystoscopy, cystogram, and upper and lower gastrointestinal series. Proving a fistulous tract may occasionally be difficult. Having the patient ingest granulated charcoal by mouth is sometimes helpful if the charcoal is subsequently found in the patient's urine. Another trick is to centrifuge the patient's urine after a barium study and x-ray the sediment, looking for minute amounts of barium. The treatment is surgical separation and closure of the fistula and primary resection of the intestinal disease. Pneumaturia alone may occasionally occur secondary to UTI with yeast or *Escherichia coli*, which ferment glucose to CO_2 and H_2O, especially in diabetics. Emphysematous cystitis may be noted in this setting.

WORKUP

The most valuable data in evaluating a patient who presents with LUTS are gained from the history and urinalysis.

History

Determine the onset and duration of symptoms and the presence of any associated symptoms. Attempt to quantify the patient's symptoms (e.g., "How many times do you awake from sleep each night to urinate?" "What is the interval between successive urinations during the daytime—every hour, every 2 hours, every 3 hours?"). Quantification of LUTS in males using the International Prostate Symptom Score (see Chapter 19) is recommended. Inquire about a history of perineal or pelvic trauma and/or prior urologic instrumentation. Note any medications that can affect urination [e.g., α-agonists, such as phenylephrine (Neo-Synephrine), anticholinergic medications, or antidepressants]. Ask the patient to keep a voiding diary, carefully recording on paper fluid intake and voiding for a 24- to 48-hour period. This information can frequently give great insight into the patient's problem.

Physical Examination

The physical examination is generally of little help in differentiating causes of obstruction. Prostatic enlargement on DRE suggests BPH as the cause; however, a normal-sized prostate does not rule out BPH. Palpate the lower abdomen for the presence of a full bladder. Examine the external genitalia, paying particular attention to the urethral meatus.

Urinalysis

Hematuria suggests a tumor, BPH, stone, or foreign body. Pyuria is also noted with the presence of stones or foreign bodies, in addition to infectious etiologies such as acute prostatitis. If infection is suspected, a urine culture should be obtained.

Uroflowmetry

Measuring the peak urine flow rate will give objective documentation of the severity of obstruction and can be valuable for following the progression of disease or response to treatment. Postvoid residual urine should always be determined following the uroflow test, generally by ultrasound bladder scan or urethral catheterization.

Cystourethroscopy

Visualization of the urethra and bladder is the single best method to assess BOO.

Chapter 3

Abnormal Prostate-Specific Antigen or Digital Rectal Examination

An abnormal or elevated level of prostate-specific antigen (PSA) is one of the most frequent reasons for urologic referral. PSA screening is used to detect early prostate cancer. Men between age 50 and 70 years should have a serum PSA and digital rectal examination (DRE) yearly. Men with a family history of prostate cancer should begin screening at age 40 years or younger. The normal range for PSA is up to 4.0 ng/mL (using the Tandem R assay).

Patients are often referred for urologic consultation because of some abnormality noted on routine DRE. The DRE is an important part of every physical examination and deserves special attention. Twenty-five percent of men with prostate cancer have normal PSA levels of less than 4.0 ng/mL. The combination of a DRE and serum PSA is the best screening method for early detection of prostate cancer. The primary function of the DRE in men is to detect prostate cancer. The size of the prostate noted on DRE correlates poorly with obstructive voiding symptoms and thus should not be used to screen for or rule out benign prostatic hyperplasia.

PROSTATE-SPECIFIC ANTIGEN

The prostate is an exocrine gland and PSA is produced by both normal and malignant prostate cells. PSA is normally disposed of through the prostatic ducts and urethra in the semen. Normally, only small amounts of PSA diffuse back into the circulation. PSA elevations occur as a result of disruption of the normal glandular structure of the prostate that allows PSA to diffuse back into the prostatic circulation, as occurs with cancer. An elevated PSA level above 4.0 ng/mL suggests the presence of prostate cancer. However, PSA elevations are not specific for cancer. PSA can be elevated in the presence of prostatitis; with an enlarged prostate;

or after lower urinary tract instrumentation, prostate biopsy, or surgery. Bicycling has also been shown to elevate PSA. A routine DRE, however, does not cause falsely elevated PSA values. An abnormal PSA level, in the absence of any of the preceding circumstances, warrants transrectal ultrasound-guided prostate biopsy. PSA measurement should be avoided if urinary tract infection is suspected.

Measurement of PSA has the highest positive predictive value of any test for prostate cancer. The positive predictive value for PSA of greater than 10 ng/mL is approximately 60%, and for PSA between 4.0 and 10 ng/mL it is approximately 20%. PSA sensitivity can be enhanced with age-specific normal values and PSA velocity to improve early detection. PSA specificity can be enhanced by PSA density and percent free PSA measurements. PSA specificity enhancements are generally used only after the first negative prostate biopsy to help determine the need for further prostate biopsies.

Age-Specific Prostate-Specific Antigen

The normal PSA level changes with age. Age-specific ranges for PSA follow: men up to age 50 years, 0 to 2.5 ng/mL; men aged 50 to 60 years, 0 to 3.5 ng/mL; and men older than 60 years, 0 to 4.0 ng/mL.

Prostate-Specific Antigen Velocity

The rate of increase of PSA over time is greater for men with prostate cancer than for men without. It has been observed that a PSA velocity of 0.75 ng/mL per year or higher is predictive of clinical prostate cancer. Obtaining at least three repeated PSA measurements over a minimum follow-up of 18 months has been suggested for PSA velocity determinations to be useful.

Prostate-Specific Antigen Density

PSA density (PSAD) is a measure of the serum PSA divided by the prostate volume. PSAD is an attempt to normalize the PSA value to the volume of the prostate because PSA level is roughly proportional to the volume of benign prostatic hyperplasia. Prostate volume must be measured by transrectal ultrasound. A PSAD of greater than 0.15 suggests cancer.

Percent Free Prostate-Specific Antigen

Most serum PSA is bound to α_1-antichymotrypsin and α_2-macroglobulin, whereas the smallest portion is in the free form. Levels of free PSA are higher in men *without* prostate cancer, and the level of complexed PSA bound to serum proteins is greater in men with malignancy. The ratio of free PSA to total PSA is higher in men with benign histology and lower in men with prostate cancer. The cut-off point for the ratio of free PSA to total PSA (approximately 18%) may differ between assays; therefore, check the specific assay for the correct values. Percent free PSA measurement is currently only recommended in men with at least one negative biopsy and a total PSA between 4.0 and 10.0 ng/mL.

Complexed Prostate-Specific Antigen

The complexed PSA assay (Immuno-1 Bayer) measures PSA bound to α_1-antichymotrypsin, which has been demonstrated to be higher in men with malignancy. In early studies, the complexed PSA assay has shown enhanced specificity over total PSA, without loss of sensitivity.

DIGITAL RECTAL EXAMINATION

The DRE should be gently performed with a well-lubricated, gloved index finger. The patient can be in a knee-chest position on his side (lateral decubitus position) or knees, or he can bend over while standing. The finger is slowly inserted into the anus until the prostate can be palpated. The prostate gland should be palpated in a systematic manner, paying careful attention to its size, shape, and consistency. Any irregularities should be noted, particularly firm or hard areas. The normal prostate gland is the size and shape of a chestnut with a rubbery consistency similar to the cartilage at the end of the nose. It can take hundreds of prostate examinations before enough experience is gained to confidently differentiate a normal from an abnormal gland. Findings and what they suggest include the following:

Nodules—nontender firm or hard nodules are highly suggestive of prostate cancer and must be biopsied.

Irregularities—markedly irregular areas, especially if firm or hard, suggest prostate cancer and should be biopsied.

Indistinct borders—loss of the normal border contours, or the impression that the gland is adherent to the pelvic sidewall, suggests prostate cancer.

Tenderness—marked tenderness to palpation with swelling suggests prostatitis.

Fluctuant—fluctuant areas associated with tenderness should suggest acute prostatitis complicated by prostatic abscess.

Crepitus—a crunchy sensation during palpation occurs in chronic prostatitis when large prostatic stones are present.

WORKUP

A PSA level above 4.0 ng/mL (or above age-specific levels) in the absence of infection, or an abnormal DRE suggestive of prostate cancer, warrants prostate needle biopsy. The continued importance of DRE is based on the fact that 25% of men with prostate cancer have a normal PSA level (<4.0 ng/mL). Transrectal ultrasound is only performed to enhance needle placement accuracy and has no inherent ability to distinguish between benign and malignant prostate tissue. If prostatitis is suspected as the cause of an abnormal PSA, then antibiotic therapy should be instituted for 4 to 6 weeks and the PSA retested.

A negative prostate biopsy does not rule out prostate cancer. A repeat PSA measurement should be made in 3 months and at regular intervals thereafter. If subsequent PSA levels remain high or are rising, careful consideration should be given to repeat the biopsy. The percent free PSA and PSA density can be helpful in this setting to enhance PSA specificity. Repeat biopsy should be considered when high-grade prostatic intraepithelial neoplasia is found on needle biopsy. There is a 30% to 50% risk of finding carcinoma on subsequent biopsies in the setting of high-grade prostatic intraepithelial neoplasia.

Hematuria

Hematuria, whether microscopic or gross, is a red flag that demands careful evaluation and must not be ignored. It is the most common presenting sign of urinary tract cancer and parenchymal renal disease. Because of the seriousness of missing a diagnosis of cancer, most urologists have a low threshold for working up any significant hematuria.

SIGNIFICANT HEMATURIA

As few as three red blood cells (RBCs) per high power field (hpf) in a voided specimen from an adult male is considered significant. RBCs found in the urine can be differentiated into two types based on origin: epithelial RBCs and glomerular RBCs.

Epithelial RBCs are regular, with smooth, rounded, or crenated membranes and an even hemoglobin distribution. As few as one epithelial RBC per hpf is abnormal and is considered a sign of urologic disease.

Glomerular RBCs are dysmorphic with irregular shapes and cell membranes and minimal or uneven hemoglobin distribution. More than 1 million RBCs normally escape from the glomerular capillaries into the urine every 24 hours. The cells become dysmorphic because of the osmotic stresses experienced during passage through the nephron. A level of more than 2 RBCs per hpf is abnormal and suggests glomerular disease.

DIFFERENTIAL DIAGNOSIS

Qualifying the type of hematuria and any associated symptoms can narrow the differential diagnosis of hematuria. Bright red gross, or macroscopic, hematuria is usually of lower urinary tract origin, whereas renal parenchymal bleeding is usually smoky, hazy, or reddish-brown owing to the formation of acid hematin in urine of low pH. Proteinuria out of proportion to the degree of hematuria (i.e.,

>2+ protein on dipstick or >1 g/24-hour urine with microscopic hematuria) suggests a renal parenchymal origin (e.g., glomerulonephritis). An active urine sediment (e.g., red cell casts or granular casts) also suggests a renal parenchymal origin. *Medical hematuria* (e.g., renal parenchymal disease excluding tumors) is suggested by the presence of glomerular RBCs, an active urinary sediment, and significant proteinuria. *Surgical hematuria* is suggested by epithelial RBCs, no casts, and minimal proteinuria.

Major Diagnosis Groups

- Cancer
- Infection
- Stones
- Benign prostatic hyperplasia
- Renal parenchymal lesions
- Trauma
- Benign idiopathic hematuria

WORKUP

History

Silent or painless hematuria suggests tumor or renal parenchymal disease. Irritative voiding symptoms (e.g., frequency, urgency, dysuria) suggest infection; however, a bladder tumor should be suspected if cultures are negative. Colicky pain suggests stone passage or sloughed renal papillae. Ask about onset and duration; associated pain; a history of trauma; and family history of diabetes, sickle cell disease, polycystic disease, or renal stones. Cyclic hematuria occurring with menses in females suggests endometriosis. Hematospermia is generally insignificant in young males; however, it can be associated with carcinoma of the prostate involving the seminal vesicle in older men. Initial hematuria suggests anterior urethral bleeding, whereas terminal hematuria is more consistent with posterior urethral bleeding (e.g., prostate or bladder neck). Total hematuria indicates bleeding at the level of the bladder or above.

Physical Examination

Fever of higher than 101°F strongly suggests a serious infection (e.g., pyelonephritis or prostatitis). Palpate the abdomen for evidence of a mass. A palpable kidney suggests tumor or hydronephrosis. A palpable bladder may indicate obstruction or retention. An irregular heart rate (from atrial fibrillation) associated with flank pain and hematuria should raise the possibility of renal embolic infarction.

Urinalysis

The urinalysis is a critical part of every workup. Differentiation of the type of hematuria (i.e., epithelial vs. glomerular) is best made using a phase contrast microscope; however, lowering the condenser on any microscope usually produces enough contrast to make the differentiation. The presence of white cells suggests an inflammatory process (e.g., infection, foreign body reaction, interstitial nephritis). The presence of casts and proteinuria suggests a medical renal parenchymal disease.

Urine Culture

A urine culture should be performed if significant pyuria or bacteriuria is present. Persistent isolated pyuria with negative cultures raises the question of tuberculosis.

Twenty-Four Hour Urine for Protein

The presence of proteinuria out of proportion to the degree of hematuria demonstrated by dipstick (i.e., >2+ protein with microhematuria) or a primary picture of glomerular bleeding should be followed by a 24-hour urine collection for quantitative protein.

Complete Blood Count

A complete blood count to detect the presence of anemia or leukocytosis should be considered.

Chemistries

Routine screening chemistries [sodium (Na), potassium (K), chloride (Cl), carbon dioxide (CO_2), blood urea nitrogen (BUN), creatinine, glucose, albumin] should be performed to evaluate renal function and look for electrolyte abnormalities. A serum albumin should be conducted only if significant protein-uria is in question.

Intravenous Urogram

An intravenous urogram is a fundamental diagnostic test for a patient with surgical hematuria. It should generally be obtained before cystoscopy if the upper tracts need further delineation by retrograde ureteropyelography.

Computed Tomography Scan of Kidneys

A computed tomography (CT) scan of the kidneys should be performed first without intravenous contrast, followed by a scan with contrast. Renal parenchymal tumors are best identified by contrast-enhanced CT.

Cystoscopy

Cystoscopy is mandatory to fully evaluate surgical hematuria. Small bladder tumors are easily missed on the cystogram phase of the intravenous urogram (IVU) or pelvic CT scan.

Renal Biopsy

Renal biopsy is indicated for patients with evidence of medical renal parenchymal disease, abnormal renal function, and protein-uria in excess of 250 mg/day.

ACUTE MANAGEMENT OF SEVERE BLADDER HEMORRHAGE

Occasionally, patients will present with severe, intractable gross hematuria that must be controlled on an acute basis. Two of the most common causes are as follows:

- Advanced bladder cancer. Patients may present with major intravesical bleeding from the tumor. The steady blood loss with slowly dropping hematocrit may necessitate transfusions, and clot formation in the bladder may cause retention.
- Hemorrhagic cystitis secondary to cyclophosphamide chemotherapy and/or radiation.

Treatment Options

1. Place a 22 to 26 F urethral catheter and hand irrigate with normal saline.
2. Start continuous bladder irrigation via a three-way Foley catheter (22–26 F) if active bleeding is minor.
3. If there is still significant active bleeding, perform cystoscopy. If there is a resectable bladder tumor, resect it. If the tumor is unresectable, attempt to coagulate any obvious areas of active bleeding.
4. Continuously irrigate intravesically with 1% alum (aluminum potassium sulfate) solution as needed.
5. Instill 1% silver nitrate solution intravesically.
6. Instill 1% to 4% formalin intravesically. (Note: formalin instillation is accompanied by a high complication rate and requires anesthesia; thus, it should be used only for serious bleeding that has failed more conservative modalities. It is contraindicated in the presence of vesicoureteral reflux; therefore, a voiding cystourethrogram must be obtained first.)
7. Embolize or ligate the iliac arteries and perform cystectomy.

5 Incontinence

Involuntary loss of urine is a frequent presenting complaint to the urologist. What constitutes significant loss can be defined by the degree of psychosocial impairment or by more objective evidence, such as the number of pads used per day. A detailed history will usually lead toward the correct diagnosis and will require only a few confirmatory tests. As with any voiding disorder (see Chapter 21), incontinence can be approached using the Wein classification as either a failure to store or a failure to empty. The major categories of incontinence follow.

TYPES OF INCONTINENCE

Total Incontinence

Total incontinence is characterized by the constant or periodic loss of urine without normal voiding and no postvoid residual. It can be thought of as a true "leak in the tank." Causes include major sphincteric abnormalities such as those that occur with exstrophy of the bladder or epispadias and abnormal anatomic connections such as those that occur with vesicovaginal fistulas or ectopic ureteral orifices.

Stress Incontinence

Stress incontinence is characterized by the involuntary loss of urine not caused by bladder contraction and is associated with physical activities such as coughing, laughing, sneezing, lifting, or exercise. This usually occurs in females with weakened pelvic floor support, urethral hypermobility, and descensus of the bladder neck. It is often associated with multiple vaginal deliveries. The net result is a loss of the normal transmission of intraabdominal pressures to the proximal urethra. Increased intraabdominal pressures will therefore cause only elevated intravesical pressures and loss of urine because the outlet resistance is unchanged. The cystometrogram is usually normal.

Urgency Incontinence

Urgency incontinence is the result of an involuntary rise in intravesical pressure secondary to bladder contraction, which overcomes outlet resistance. Bladder instability or hyperreflexia generally produces a sensation of urgency of urination in most patients; however, it can present with incontinence alone. Common causes of detrusor instability include loss of cortical inhibition of the voiding reflex (e.g., those that occur after strokes or dementia or with parkinsonism). However, the more common local causes of detrusor instability, such as infection, bladder stone, tumor (carcinoma in situ), interstitial cystitis, or foreign body, must always be ruled out first.

Overflow Incontinence

Overflow incontinence is said to be paradoxical because urine loss is the result of a failure of the bladder to empty, rather than an inability to properly store urine. Causes include bladder outlet obstruction, detrusor weakness, or a combination. Males with outlet obstruction secondary to benign prostatic hyperplasia or strictures typically present with symptoms of frequency; slow, weak stream; and voiding small volumes. The hallmark of overflow incontinence is a high postvoid urine volume. Females more typically have detrusor hypotonicity with poor emptying and high residuals secondary to diabetes mellitus, autonomic neuropathy, or anticholinergic medications (e.g., tranquilizers).

Enuresis

Enuresis refers to involuntary wetting in children. It is generally a problem at night and should be referred to as nocturnal enuresis as opposed to diurnal enuresis. However, these qualifiers are often omitted, and enuresis is usually taken to mean bedwetting. Enuresis is a common problem and should be viewed as a developmental lag in the inhibitory influence of the central nervous system on the urinary bladder. However, behavioral or stress factors are believed also to be involved in some children. Twelve percent of 6-year-olds, 3% of 12-year-olds, and 1% of 18-year-olds wet their beds.

Primary enuretics are children who have been wet since birth, whereas *secondary enuretics* have had a period of dryness before reverting to wetting. Most primary enuresis resolves by the second or third year of life; however, some children will continue to wet into later years. No objective organic lesion will be identified in the true enuretic other than a lower functional bladder capacity. The most characteristic trait of enuretics is their sound sleeping habits. The diagnosis is made by excluding urologic disease that could be responsible (e.g., urinary tract infections, reflux, meatal stenosis, bladder outlet obstruction, or neurologic disease). A careful history, urinalysis, and plain film of the abdomen are generally sufficient to work up the enuretic child. If the history or urinalysis suggests organic disease, then a more thorough investigation, including voiding cystourethrogram (VCUG), intravenous urography, and cystoscopy, is in order.

Spontaneous resolution can be expected with regularity, requiring only parental reassurance, toilet training, and fluid restriction before bedtime. More aggressive measures should be considered in the child reaching school age.

DIAGNOSIS

History

A good voiding history is essential and will often reveal the correct diagnosis without the need for an elaborate evaluation. Inquire about specific details of symptoms, including urgency, frequency, dysuria, stress leakage, and times of leakage. A detailed history of other medical problems, including all medications, surgical history, and parity, is important. Note caffeine intake. Ask if the patient uses protection and, if so, how many pads per day are needed. A voiding diary can be helpful.

Physical Examination

Abdominal, pelvic, and rectal examinations should be routine, along with a neurologic assessment. Note any masses, cystoceles, rectoceles, rectal sphincter tone, fecal impaction, or evidence of estrogen deficiency in females. A "Q-tip test" can be performed to test for pelvic floor relaxation in women.

Laboratory Studies

Urinalysis, urine culture, serum electrolytes, blood urea nitrogen (BUN), creatinine, and fasting blood sugar should be obtained. Atypical vaginal cultures may be productive in difficult cases of overactive bladder.

Postvoid Residual Urine

Measurement of postvoid residual urine (PVR) is probably the single most useful piece of information in understanding incontinence. It helps categorize the disorder as failure to store or failure to empty.

Urodynamics

Urodynamic studies, including uroflow and cystometry, should be obtained when indicated. Abdominal leak point pressure measurement can identify intrinsic sphincter dysfunction.

X-Ray Studies

A VCUG is often helpful, particularly in patients with suspected stress urinary incontinence. Bladder descensus with cystocele can be readily appreciated. An intravenous urogram is indicated in patients with hematuria, persistent infections, or suspected tumor.

Cystoscopy

Cystoscopy can be reserved for patients with hematuria, persistent infections, suspected tumor, or a history of prior surgical intervention.

MANAGEMENT

Stress Incontinence

Intraurethral and bladder neck injections with collagen can give short-term improvement. Retropubic slings and suspensions, pubovaginal sling procedures and transvaginal suspensions, vaginal pessaries, α-adrenergic stimulation to increase bladder outlet resistance (ephedrine or phenylpropanolamine), or estrogen therapy to increase α-adrenergic receptor sensitivity in the bladder neck and proximal urethra can be used (0.5 g Estrace vaginal cream on Monday, Wednesday, and Friday).

Urgency Incontinence (Detrusor Instability)

Pharmacotherapy (oxybutynin, tolterodine, solifenacin, trospium, darifenacin), bladder denervation, and augmentation cystoplasty are treatment options.

Overflow Incontinence

Intermittent self-catheterization is appropriate for patients with bladder atony. Males with outlet resistance should benefit from surgical relief of the obstruction if detrusor function can be salvaged. Indwelling urethral catheters should be avoided if possible. Intermittent self-catheterization would be preferable.

Total Incontinence

Patients with documented anatomic problems such as exstrophy, epispadias, ectopic ureters, or fistulas will require appropriate surgical intervention. Artificial urinary sphincters may be necessary in some instances.

Enuresis

True enuresis will generally resolve spontaneously between age 2 and 6 years. Objective urologic disease must be ruled out if suspected. Alarm conditioning and pharmacotherapy may be necessary. Pharmacologic therapy includes imipramine [Tofranil 25 mg orally (PO) at bedtime] or oxybutynin (Ditropan 5 mg PO at bedtime). Intranasal or oral arginine vasopressin [DDAVP 20 μg at bedtime (qhs)] can be tried in children age 6 years or older.

6 Acute Stone Management

PRESENTATION

The patient with stone typically presents with unilateral renal colic and hematuria. Renal colic refers to an intermittent flank pain arising in the kidney or ureter and may radiate to the ipsilateral groin or testis. Patients generally toss about and cannot find a comfortable position. Guarding with nausea and vomiting is occasionally noted. Low-grade fever and mild elevation of the white blood cell count may be present. Evidence of serious infection (e.g., high-grade fever, white count, and pyuria) demands immediate intervention, especially in diabetics.

DIAGNOSIS

Urinalysis will almost always show red blood cells, and 90% of stones can be demonstrated on a kidney, ureter, and bladder (KUB) film of the abdomen. If a stone is seen on KUB, then the intravenous urogram (IVU) need not be obtained immediately. A thorough bowel preparation and a high-quality nonemergent study will yield more information. A stone protocol (non-contrast) computed tomography (CT) scan has become the standard initial workup of patients with suspected stone. However, if high-grade obstruction requiring acute intervention is suspected, then an emergency IVU should be obtained.

Workup

■ Laboratory Tests

A urinalysis should always be obtained. Hematuria will be present in most cases. Pyuria would suggest an associated infection that will need immediate attention. A urine culture should be ordered if the urinalysis indicates pyuria or significant bacteriuria. A serum creatinine level should be obtained to evaluate renal function. A complete blood count may be indicated to screen for evidence of serious infection.

■ Imaging Studies

A noncontrast CT scan of the abdomen and pelvis using a stone protocol has replaced the standard IVU in the initial workup for acute stone in most emergency room settings. Its advantages are speed, no need for intravenous contrast or monitoring, and the ability to identify even small radiolucent uric acid stones. A negative CT is strong evidence against the presence of a stone. However, CT can be a poor indicator of the degree of obstruction and hydronephrosis. An IVU may still be useful if the severity of obstruction is in question.

MANAGEMENT

Immediate care of the patient with acute stone is based on the following considerations:
1. Size and location of the stone and likelihood of its passing spontaneously
2. Any complicating medical problems (e.g., diabetes or solitary kidney)
3. Complications related to the stone (e.g., high-grade obstruction or infection)

Indications for Hospitalization

1. High-grade obstruction, especially when associated with stones greater than 10 mm, will require early intervention (i.e., ureteral stents or percutaneous nephrostomy).
2. High fever (>101°F) suggests pyelonephritis is present, and appropriate antibiotics should be started immediately.
3. Patients with uncontrollable pain requiring parenteral analgesics should be hospitalized.
4. Patients with severe nausea with dehydration requiring intravenous fluids should be hospitalized.
5. Patients with a single functioning kidney at risk of acute renal failure require hospitalization.

Diabetics

The diabetic patient with acute stone disease has an increased risk of developing complications (e.g., infection and contrast-mediated nephrotoxicity). This is especially true for insulin-dependent diabetics out of control. Hospitalization is often indicated. Caution is indicated when intravenous contrast is given to diabetics on metformin (Glucophage). Metformin should be discontinued for 48 hours after intravenous iodinated contrast is used. Nonionic, iso-osmolar contrast should be used whenever possible.

Pregnancy

Pregnant woman who present with renal colic and microscopic hematuria should undergo renal ultrasound. If hydronephrosis is present, presumption of a ureteral calculus can be made. If renal colic fails to resolve with hydration and analgesics or in the setting of severe obstruction or sepsis, then retrograde placement of a silicone double-J ureteral stent under local anesthesia is a reasonable course.

Extracorporeal Shock Wave Lithotripsy Treatment

Patients who have had recent extracorporeal shock wave lithotripsy (ESWL) may present with renal colic owing to passing stone fragments (Steinstrasse). Stent placement *may* be necessary.

Inpatient

Patients admitted for acute stone management should receive vigorous fluid resuscitation, especially the diabetic with infection. Antibiotics should be given as indicated. High-grade obstruction should be relieved with placement of a retrograde ureteral stent or percutaneous nephrostomy. Urine should be strained for stones.

Outpatient Management

For the otherwise healthy individual with an acute stone less than 5 mm in diameter, outpatient management is appropriate. Patients should be instructed to drink plenty of fluids, strain the urine to catch the stone, and save the stone for analysis. They should be given an adequate supply of oral analgesics. Follow-up should include a weekly or biweekly KUB to monitor progress of the stone passage. Patients with stones between 5 and 10 mm are less likely to pass the stone spontaneously and should be considered for early elective intervention in the absence of other complicating factors (e.g., infection, high-grade obstruction, or solitary kidney). Stones that are larger than 10 mm will rarely pass.

PAPILLARY NECROSIS

Papillary necrosis is the result of toxic or ischemic injury to the papillary tip with subsequent necrosis. It is most commonly associated with analgesic abuse, pyelonephritis in diabetics, sickle cell disease, and systemic vasculitis in middle-aged women. Rarely will patients present with renal colic and hematuria (similar to an obstructing stone) secondary to acute sloughing of necrotic papillae with ureteral obstruction. Most patients will present with insidious onset of renal failure. An intravenous pyelogram (IVP) will show calyceal irregularities or ring shadows around sloughed papilla within the calyx. Fragments of the papillae may be found in the urinary sediment. The sloughed papillae can cause obstruction or serve as a nidus for persistent infection. Management consists of treating infection, relieving obstruction, and removing causative agents (analgesics).

Genitourinary Pain

The process of diagnosing the etiology of a patient's pain is still one of the most difficult aspects of clinical medicine. Here, probably more than anywhere else, clinical experience and judgment are vital elements. I recommend *Cope's Early Diagnosis of the Acute Abdomen* by William Silen (New York: Oxford University Press, 2005). It is an unequaled crash course in clinical experience and judgment.

KIDNEY PAIN

Pain associated with the kidney is the result of sudden distention of the renal capsule, as occurs with acute ureteral obstruction. It is referred to as flank pain and is usually colicky in nature (i.e., intermittent or in waves). Patients are often restless and cannot find a comfortable position. Reflex nausea and vomiting *may* be noted because of the common autonomic and sensory innervation of the gastrointestinal and urologic systems.

A dull, constant ache in the costovertebral angle also can characterize renal pain. This is less likely to be associated with acute obstruction but rather is secondary to renal parenchymal enlargement from pyelonephritis or a tumor. Renal pain must not be confused with flank or back pain of musculoskeletal origin or radiculitis, which can be aggravated or relieved by postural changes. Finally, remember that many renal diseases are painless, despite massive degrees of obstruction or kidney enlargement by tumors, because of the slow, gradual progression of the disease.

URETERAL PAIN

Ureteral pain also is colicky and is intimately related to renal pain. Acute ureteral obstruction, as with a stone, will cause hyperperistalsis and spasm of the ureteral smooth muscle as it attempts to overcome the obstruction. Flank pain from renal capsular distention also will be noted, and the pain will radiate from the flank down the ipsilateral lower quadrant into the scrotum and testicle in male patients or the vulva in female patients. The level of ureteral obstruction can often be inferred by how far into the groin the pain radiates. Always be careful not to overlook other common intraabdominal pathology, such as appendicitis and diverticulitis, which can often be confused with ureteral pain.

BLADDER PAIN

Overdistention of the bladder as with acute urinary retention can produce severe suprapubic pain. However, most bladder pathology manifests with lower urinary tract symptoms (see Chapter 2), such as frequency, urgency, and dysuria, rather than suprapubic pain. Diseases of the uterus, such as fibroids and endometriosis, or of the colon, such as inflammation or fecal impaction, also may first be seen with suprapubic pain.

PROSTATIC PAIN

Inflammatory conditions of the prostate can appear with a vague discomfort or fullness in the perineal or rectal area; however, lower urinary tract symptoms are usually the primary complaint. Prostate cancer will rarely cause pain in the perineal area until an advanced stage.

TESTICULAR PAIN

Testicular pain, as will occur with torsion, epididymo-orchitis, or trauma, is primarily felt locally in the area of the testicle and epididymis and may radiate to the ipsilateral lower abdomen (see Chapter 10). Testis cancer is typically painless.

BACK AND LEG PAIN

Patients with prostate cancer may occasionally first be seen with complaints of low back pain radiating down one or both legs, secondary to bony metastases. Any evidence of lower-extremity weakness or difficulty walking should alert one to the possibility of cord or nerve root compression and must be treated as a medical emergency (see Chapter 22). Lower urinary tract symptoms are often associated with low back pain.

Erectile Dysfunction

Erectile dysfunction (ED), defined as the inability to maintain an erect penis with sufficient rigidity for sexual intercourse, is an increasingly common presenting complaint and is estimated to affect 10 million men in the United States. ED can include partial or brief erections to complete ED (impotence). With basic knowledge about the physiology and neuropharmacology of erection, we can approach the problems systematically and logically.

PHYSIOLOGY

In brief, the neurovascular mechanism of erection involves the following. In the flaccid state, cavernosal smooth muscle tone is high, causing an increased resistance to incoming blood. Erection occurs via stimulation by parasympathetic fibers of the pelvic plexus and cavernous nerves. Resulting arteriolar dilation and sinusoidal smooth muscle relaxation within the corpora cavernosa allow increased arterial blood flow. As the cavernosal sinusoids distend with incoming blood, the subtunical venular plexuses become compressed, thus reducing venous outflow. With stretching of the tunica albuginea to its capacity, the emissary veins eventually close within the tunical layers, further decreasing venous outflow to a minimum. The direct inducer of sinusoidal smooth muscle relaxation has been identified as endothelium-derived relaxing factor, now known to be nitric oxide, by way of its action on cyclic guanosine monophosphate (cGMP). Tonic sinusoidal smooth muscle contraction of the normally flaccid penis may be mediated by the neurotransmitter endothelin-1. Thus physiologic erections are the result of nitric oxide–induced cGMP. cGMP is broken down by the enzyme phosphodiesterase type 5 (PD-5).

PHARMACOLOGY

Some drugs known to produce erections include papaverine, nitroglycerin, α-blockers such as phentolamine, prostaglandin

E_1 (PGE$_1$), and PD-5 inhibitors. Some drugs known to cause detumescence include epinephrine, norepinephrine, phenylephrine, dopamine, and metaraminol.

ETIOLOGY

Psychogenic

Psychological causes (e.g., performance anxiety, depression) used to be considered the most common reason for ED but are now thought to be the primary factors in only a few cases. Secondary psychological components can be expected in all cases.

Organic (50%–90%)

- *Vasculogenic.* This is the most common single cause and is due to either poor inflow (e.g., arterial insufficiency, large-vessel atherosclerosis, or small-vessel diabetes) or enhanced outflow (e.g., venous leak).
- *Endocrine.* Hypogonadotropic males with small atrophic testes and low serum testosterone levels.
- *Neurologic.* Common neurologic etiologies include diabetic neuropathy, spinal cord injury, and development after surgery.
- *End-organ failure.* Priapism or Peyronie's disease can cause cavernosal injury, which can result in ED.

Iatrogenic

- *Medications.* Drug-induced impotence was reported to constitute 25% of cases in one review. Patients taking medications affecting the autonomic nervous system or vascular systems may benefit from attempts to change or modify these medications; however, modification is frequently neither successful nor an option because of the patient's poor cardiovascular status. Alcoholism, a common cause of impotence, may result in decreased testosterone and increased estrogen levels and alcoholic polyneuropathy. Cigarette smoking may induce vasoconstriction and sinusoidal smooth muscle contraction. Psychotropic agents such as phenothiazines, butyrophenones, tricyclic antidepressants, and monoamine oxidase inhibitors have been implicated in ED.

- *Pelvic surgery*. Damage to pelvic nerves or pudendal arteries during pelvic surgery (e.g., after a radical prostatectomy, cystectomy, or abdominal perineal resection) can result in ED.

WORKUP

History and Physical Examination

Question patients concerning recent life crises such as deaths, divorce, financial problems, or loss of job. Determine whether the patient ever has an erection (e.g., on arising in the morning) and when his last normal erection was. Take a careful drug history, including alcohol, tobacco, and illegal drugs. Question for evidence of vascular disease (e.g., claudication, coronary artery disease, hypertension, or diabetes). Ask about a history of pelvic or perineal trauma or surgery. Examination should include evidence of secondary sexual characteristics, peripheral pulses, neurologic examination, and general genitourinary examination, with attention to possible plaques along the shaft of the penis (i.e., Peyronie's disease; see Chapter 9).

Laboratory Tests

- Fasting blood glucose—screening for diabetes
- Serum free testosterone (hypogonadism) and prolactin (hyperprolactinemia) levels

Special Studies

- Penile rigidity monitoring gives an objective, noninvasive assessment of both tumescence and rigidity.
- Vasoactive intracavernous injection. The ability to have a full erection within 10 to 15 minutes of an intracavernous papaverine or PGE_1 injection essentially eliminates significant arterial or venous impairment. Further vascular evaluation is probably unnecessary.
- Duplex ultrasound and color Doppler analysis (before and after papaverine injection) evaluates cavernosal anatomy and artery flow.
- Dynamic cavernosography and cavernosometry. Monitoring intracavernous pressures while performing corpora

cavernosography during an artificial erection (e.g., induced by papaverine or saline perfusion) is used to evaluate the penile veins for a leak.

- Pudendal arteriography (after papaverine injection) has been used to evaluate posttraumatic impotence.

TREATMENT

The introduction of oral PD-5 inhibitors has revolutionized the workup and management of ED. PD-5 inhibitors have generally replaced the use of specialized studies in most men with ED. A trial of a PD-5 inhibitor is often the first approach in men without contraindications to these agents.

Phosphodiesterase-5 Inhibitors

PD-5 inhibitors enhance the effects of nitric oxide–activated increases in cGMP by inhibiting the breakdown of cGMP. PD-5 inhibitors are contraindicated in patients taking nitrates or those who have serious cardiovascular compromise. They also should be avoided or used with caution when taken with α-blockers. PD-5 inhibitors have a number of other adverse drug interactions, which must be cautioned against (refer to prescribing inserts). Common side effects include headache, flushing of the face, and upset stomach. Some of the serious side effects include myocardial infarction, stroke, and loss of vision. PD-5 inhibitors should be used with caution.

Sildenafil (Viagra) was the first PD-5 inhibitor on the market. Sildenafil should be effective approximately 30 to 60 minutes after an oral dose. Dosages are 25, 50, or 100 mg.

Vardenafil (Levitra) was the second PD-5 inhibitor released. It has a shorter onset of action. Dosages are 2.5, 5, 10, or 20 mg.

Todalafil (Cialis) is the most recent PD-5 inhibitor. It boasts a longer half-life and thus may last for up to 36 hours. Dosages are 5, 10, or 20 mg.

Mechanical Vacuum Constriction Devices

External vacuum-pump devices have proven successful for many patients and are a good initial approach before more invasive modalities.

Testosterone Injections

Testosterone injections (testosterone enanthate 200 mg IM q3wk) have occasionally been shown to be effective in patients with documented low testosterone levels. Caution should be used in elderly patients suspected of having prostate cancer.

Vasoactive Intracavernous Injections

Self-administered intracavernous PGE_1 combination therapy (papaverine 12 mg/mL, PGE_1 9 μg/mL, and phentolamine 1 mg/mL) has been demonstrated to be beneficial. Complications include dizziness, flushing, hypotension, local pain, infection, hematomas, priapism, and fibrosis of the corpora cavernosa.

Psychotherapy/Sex Therapy

Referral to a sexual-dysfunction clinic is indicated for patients with a clear psychological etiology.

Vascular Surgery

Vascular causes have been treated with various procedures to either improve arterial inflow or slow venous outflow from the corpora cavernosa. These techniques have met with limited success even in highly specialized hands. Large-vessel stenosis, such as in the hypogastrics, has occasionally been treated with balloon dilatation. Isolated venous leaks have been successfully treated with vein ligation.

Penile Prostheses

Prostheses remain a form of therapy for patients with erectile impotence that cannot be managed with less invasive techniques. Success is generally good, with few complications. The most frequent complications include infection (which necessitates removal of prosthesis), erosion, and malfunction. Prostheses should be used with caution to treat patients for whom psychotherapy failed. Patients should be warned that no return to normal erection is possible once a prosthesis has been used. Be sure to correct any bladder-outlet obstruction (e.g., benign prostatic hyperplasia) before a prosthesis is inserted. Transurethral surgery can be a challenge with a penile prosthesis in place.

Penile Complaints

PRIAPISM

Priapism is an abnormally prolonged penile erection (>6 hours) that does not result from sexual desire. It generally involves only the corpora cavernosa and not the spongiosum. It is often associated with pain and difficulty urinating. It can occur at any age and may last for several days to several weeks if left untreated.

Etiology

Priapism can be classified into two distinct types: low-flow (ischemic) veno-occlusive and high-flow (nonischemic) arterial priapism. Low-flow ischemic priapism is secondary to failure of the detumescence mechanism and obstruction of the venous drainage of the corpora cavernosa. Ischemic priapism is associated with acidotic cavernosal blood gases. High-flow priapism is generally the result of trauma that causes laceration or rupture of the cavernous artery within the corpora cavernosa.

Many cases are classified as primary or idiopathic because the etiology is unknown. Other major causes of priapism include drug and alcohol abuse, erectile-dysfunction drug therapy, sickle cell disease, neoplastic diseases, and trauma. *Drugs* that affect the neurovascular or central nervous system can potentially cause priapism. These include psychotropics (e.g., chlorpromazine or trazodone), antihypertensives (especially hydralazine, guanethidine, and prazosin), and alcohol. Anticoagulants (e.g., heparin) also have been associated with cases of priapism. Pharmacologic injection therapy to treat erectile dysfunction, such as intracavernous injection of papaverine or prostaglandin E_1, have become the most common causes of priapism.

Sickle cell disease and trait are common etiologies in boys and account for about 10% to 20% of cases overall. Attacks often occur during sleep with sludging of red cells in the corpora cavernosa after a normal physiologic nocturnal erection.

Neoplastic diseases can obstruct corporal outflow. Leukemias are the most common cause of priapism in boys.

Trauma can result in priapism secondary to hematoma formation and compression of venous drainage or injury to the cavernous artery and high-flow priapism.

Diagnosis

The diagnosis of priapism is straightforward. Patients are first seen with a persistent erection (>6 hours) without sexual desire. Pain and fever may be present along with difficulty voiding. On physical examination, the corpora cavernosa are fully rigid in low-flow priapism and partially to fully rigid in high-flow priapism. The glans penis is generally flaccid. Patients will often delay seeking attention because of embarrassment. Recognition of any underlying etiology, such as neoplasm or sickle cell disease, is important because it may affect the plan of treatment. A sickle cell preparation for hemoglobin S should be performed on all black patients with priapism. A complete blood count should be obtained to rule out leukemia. A thorough drug history is essential. Intracavernosal injection therapy complications will be evident from the history. Cavernosal blood gases and duplex ultrasound scanning can be helpful in differentiating ischemic and nonischemic priapism.

Management

Priapism can result in impotence in up to 50% of cases, and early treatment can reduce but not eliminate the risk. Patients using pharmacologic injection therapy should be instructed to use pseudoephedrine, an over-the-counter decongestant, if their erection lasts longer than 4 hours, possibly to avert a more serious priapism. Conservative management in other forms of priapism is often unsuccessful; however, an initial intramuscular injection of a narcotic analgesic is reasonable. Definitive therapy should not be delayed because the risk of permanent impotence increases significantly if treatment is not started within 24 to 48 hours. Remember that the penis in priapism is usually ischemic, despite being engorged with blood, and that pain is usually a good indication that tissue ischemia has occurred. Intracorporal blood-gas determinations can be used to monitor hypoxemia and acidosis.

Treatment Options

Medical management should be exhausted before resorting to surgical treatments.

1. Aspiration of 50 to 100 mL of stagnant blood through a small needle placed directly in the corporal body or through the glans into the corpora cavernosa should be tried initially. The patient must be sedated first and the glans anesthetized with local lidocaine (Xylocaine) 1%, without epinephrine. After aspiration, gentle irrigation of the corpora with normal saline is sometimes helpful. Alternatively, the dark blood can be squeezed out until bright-red blood returns. Use of prophylactic antibiotics is recommended with aspiration.

2. After aspiration, intracavernous injection with an α-adrenergic agonist should be attempted in low-flow non–sickle cell patients. Pharmacotherapy with α-adrenergic agents is the treatment of choice for priapism secondary to intracavernous injection therapy (e.g., papaverine or prostaglandin E_1). This injection should be cautiously performed because α-agonists may prolong tissue ischemia. Aspiration of 10 to 20 mL of blood followed by injection of epinephrine (10–20 μg diluted in 1 mL normal saline) or phenylephrine (100–200 μg diluted in 1 mL normal saline) has been successful. This can be repeated every 5 minutes until detumescence occurs. A transient increase in blood pressure can be expected. Caution should be exercised in patients with a history of severe cardiac or cerebrovascular disease.

3. Oral terbutaline (5–10 mg PO) has been shown to be effective in patients with priapism secondary to intracavernous injection therapy for erectile dysfunction.

4. Patients with sickle cell disease should be treated conservatively with prompt aggressive hydration, oxygenation, and metabolic alkalinization to reduce further sickling. Aspiration and irrigation of the corpora should be performed. Transfusion and erythropheresis may be necessary.

5. Fistula creation between spongiosum of the glans and cavernosa by using a Travenol Tru-Cut biopsy needle (Winter's procedure) is a reasonable next step after failure of medical management. This will provide additional continuous drainage of the cavernosa via the corpus spongiosum.

6. Formal shunt creation may be necessary with an open surgical procedure:
   a. A side-to-side anastomotic shunt between the corpus spongiosum and cavernosum at the base of the penis may be successful;

  b. Alternatively, a saphenous vein–corpus cavernosum shunt may be necessary for difficult cases.
7. Patients with high-flow priapism may require arteriography with embolization of the internal pudendal artery.

Tight circumferential dressings around the penis should be avoided.

PHIMOSIS

Phimosis is a narrowing or constriction of the distal penile foreskin that prevents its normal retraction over the glans. Phimosis is most commonly acquired as a result of poor hygiene and chronic infection. Phimosis rarely occurs with a normal foreskin. The inability to retract the foreskin is normal during early infancy. These congenital adhesions will naturally separate during the first 1 to 2 years of life and are not an indication for circumcision. Complications of phimosis include balanitis, posthitis, paraphimosis, and penile carcinoma.

Management

Minor phimosis can be managed with hygiene alone; however, more advanced phimosis will require circumcision. If significant infection is present (balanoposthitis), an immediate dorsal slit may be necessary to provide proper drainage and to allow resolution of the infection before attempting circumcision.

PARAPHIMOSIS

In paraphimosis, the retracted foreskin remains trapped behind the glans penis, with secondary swelling, pain, and inflammation. Untreated, it can progress through major infection and eventual ischemia of the glans to gangrene. Paraphimosis is frequently the result of a partially phimotic foreskin that has been retracted and not released. It also can frequently occur in a patient with a urethral catheter in place and the foreskin retracted.

Management

An initial attempt at manual reduction should be made. The patient should first be premedicated with meperidine (Demerol) or morphine. Manual reduction is done by placing both thumbs on the glans and trapping the foreskin between the second and third fingers of each hand. The thumbs are then pushed toward the second and third fingers while pulling the foreskin over the glans. Compression of the glans also can help reduce the foreskin. Elective circumcision should be planned after swelling and inflammation have subsided. If manual reduction fails, a dorsal slit or circumcision under local anesthesia should be performed without delay.

BALANOPOSTHITIS

Balanitis refers to an inflammation of the superficial layers of the glans penis, whereas posthitis is an inflammation of the prepuce. The two conditions commonly occur together and are often associated with poor hygiene and phimosis.

Management

Meticulous hygiene is the key to treatment and prevention. Patients must be instructed to retract the foreskin several times a day for cleansing with mild soap and water and thorough drying. Local application of antibiotic ointments (e.g., Bacitracin or Neosporin) or steroid-based creams (e.g., Kenalog or Mycolog) may be beneficial. Oral antibiotics or antifungal agents [e.g., fluconazole (Diflucan)] also can aid resolution. In severe cases, a dorsal slit may be necessary to establish drainage and to allow proper cleansing. Circumcision should be considered after inflammation has subsided.

PEYRONIE'S DISEASE

Peyronie's disease is characterized by scarlike lesions of the tunica albuginea of the penis. Once thought to be a primarily inflammatory or autoimmune disease, it is now believed to be the result of trauma to the penis during sexual activity. The trauma causes collagen deposition and scar formation, resulting in curvature and functional shortening of the penis. Painful erection also is characteristic early in the disease. Erectile dysfunction is common and usually precedes the development of Peyronie's disease. Spontaneous resolution can be expected in up to 50% of patients; however, extensive plaques with calcification may not resolve.

Management

The mainstay of treatment is to discontinue trauma to the site, limiting further injury and allowing time for natural healing and resolution.

■ Medical Treatment

Many nonsurgical treatments have been tried for Peyronie's disease, most with limited success.
1. Vitamin E 400 mg twice a day PO.
2. Potassium para-aminobenzoate (Potaba) 12 g/day, in four to six divided doses, is expensive and of uncertain benefit.
3. Intralesional steroid injection is probably of little benefit and may worsen the lesions.
4. Small-dose radiation can alleviate pain but does not correct the bending deformity.
5. Other medical interventions, such as colchicine or calcium channel blockers, are unproven.

■ Surgical Treatment

Surgical intervention to correct penile curvature should be delayed for at least 1 year to allow adequate time for spontaneous resolution or medical therapy to take effect.

Scrotal Mass

Scrotal pathology is a common cause of referral to the urologist. Patients will either present with a mass in the scrotum, with or without pain, or with an empty scrotum (cryptorchidism), which is covered in the next chapter. When evaluating a scrotal mass, always work through the complete differential diagnosis. This helps avoid the significant consequences of misdiagnosing testicular torsion or tumor. A thorough understanding of each pathologic condition is the best tool for correct diagnosis.

REVIEW OF PATHOLOGY

Testicular Torsion

Torsion refers to a twisting of the testis and spermatic cord around a vertical axis, resulting in venous obstruction, progressive swelling, arterial compromise, and eventually testicular infarction. Torsion must be considered in the initial diagnosis of any scrotal pathology because without immediate detorsion, the testis will be lost. Two types of torsion occur: extravaginal and intravaginal.

■ Extravaginal Torsion

Extravaginal torsion occurs in neonates (and occasionally in utero) because of incomplete attachment of the gubernaculum and testicular tunics to the scrotal wall. This incomplete attachment leaves the testis, epididymis, and tunica vaginalis free to twist within the scrotum. Extravaginal torsion accounts for fewer than 10% of all cases of testicular torsion. Infants typically present in minimal distress with a firm, painless scrotal mass that does not transilluminate. Most of these testes will be gangrenous at exploration, and the salvage rate is poor. Early recognition of postnatal torsion is a clear indication for surgery because of the increased chance for testicular salvage. However, intrauterine torsion rarely results in testicular salvage, so the indications for surgery are less clear. Removal of the infarcted testis has been recommended by some authors because of the theoretic concern for autoimmune damage to the contralateral testis, with resultant fertility problems in the adult.

▣ Intravaginal Torsion

This condition can occur at any age but is most common among adolescents. It is the result of an abnormally narrowed testicular mesentery, with the tunica vaginalis almost completely surrounding the entire testis and epididymis. This narrowed mesentery facilitates twisting of the testis within the tunica vaginalis about its vascular pedicle and gives an appearance termed the "bell-clapper" deformity.

▣ Diagnosis

The typical patient presents with sudden onset of pain and swelling, occasionally associated with some minor trauma. The testis will be tender, is often high in the scrotum because of shortening by the twisted cord, and may have a transverse lie or an anteriorly positioned epididymis. Urinalysis is usually negative. Elevation of the scrotum will not relieve the pain (negative Prehn's sign). Color-flow Doppler ultrasonography should be obtained without hesitation and has become the test of choice. A radionuclide testicular scan may be useful in equivocal cases if performed early after the onset of symptoms and before significant reactive hyperemia of the scrotal skin occurs. Surgical exploration is the best diagnostic test and should not be delayed if this diagnosis is seriously considered.

▣ Treatment

Treatment consists of immediate detorsion. Correction within 6 hours of onset of pain usually results in a normal testis. Delay for more than 12 hours results in poor testicular salvage (~20%). Manual detorsion can be attempted by either lifting the scrotum or rotating the testis about its vascular pedicle. Successful manual detorsion must still be followed by surgical orchiopexy. An unsuccessful attempt at manual detorsion requires immediate surgical exploration. The clearly infarcted testis should be removed; however, if viability is in doubt, it should be left in situ because Leydig cell function may be preserved. After detorsion, the testis should be fixed to the scrotal wall with two to three nonabsorbable sutures to prevent repeated torsion. The contralateral testis must also be fixed because of the high incidence of its subsequent torsion.

Testicular Appendages

The five potential testicular appendages are as follows: (a) appendix testis, (b) appendix epididymis, (c) paradidymis organ of Giraldes, (d) superior Haller's vas aberrans, and (e) inferior Haller's vas aberrans. Only the appendix testis and the appendix epididymis are regularly found. Their only importance is that they also can undergo torsion and mimic testicular torsion. Torsion of the appendix testis is by far the most common and typically occurs as acute onset of scrotal pain in an adolescent. Generally, a tender, pea-sized nodule can be palpated near the upper pole of the testis. An infarcted appendage can often be seen as a small blue-black dot through the scrotal skin (blue dot sign). Color-flow Doppler ultrasound should be performed to confirm blood flow to the testis. If the diagnosis is doubtful, surgical exploration should be performed to rule out testicular torsion; otherwise, conservative management may be considered. If surgery is performed, the infarcted appendage should simply be excised.

Testicular Tumors

Testicular cancers (see Chapter 26) usually are discovered as an incidental finding of a painless lump or nodule in the scrotum of a male aged 20 to 40 years. The lump or nodule may be accompanied by a heavy sensation or dull ache in the lower abdomen. Occasionally, testis cancers present with acute pain secondary to rapid growth, with hemorrhage and necrosis. More commonly, however, they are hard, nontender nodules localized to the testis. They do not transilluminate, yet an associated hydrocele may occur. Up to 10% of testis cancers will present initially with epididymitis. Benign testicular tumors are rare (<1%) and include teratoma of childhood, epidermoid cyst, dermoid cyst, simple testicular cyst, cyst of tunica albuginea, and adenomatoid tumor. Testicular ultrasound should be performed. The pathologic diagnosis is made by radical inguinal orchiectomy. Consider all testicular masses malignant until proven otherwise.

Inguinal Hernia

An inguinal hernia often is first seen as a scrotal mass secondary to loops of bowel within the scrotum. Indirect inguinal hernias may be secondary to a patent processus vaginalis or protrusion of a new peritoneal process following the same path along the cord into the scrotum. Direct inguinal hernias result from weakness of the transversalis fascia at Hesselbach's triangle, with peritoneal outpouching into the area of the external ring only, rarely descending into the scrotum. An inguinal hernia that cannot be reduced is said to be incarcerated. If the vascular supply of the herniated organ (usually bowel) is compromised, it is said to be strangulated—a surgical emergency.

Epididymitis

Acute epididymitis may present in any age group as sudden onset of pain and swelling in the scrotum (refer to Chapter 17). Urinalysis is usually positive for inflammatory cells, and temperature is often elevated. A urethral discharge or irritative voiding symptoms are common. Elevation of the scrotum may decrease the patient's pain (positive Prehn's sign). Early, the swelling and tenderness can often be localized to the tail of the epididymis; however, this distinction blurs as the infection progresses. An inflammatory hydrocele may develop within a few days. Fixation of the testicle to the scrotal wall suggests abscess formation. Color-flow Doppler testicular ultrasound can help make the diagnosis by demonstrating increased blood flow.

Hydrocele

A hydrocele is a fluid collection within the tunica vaginalis surrounding the testis. It presents as a painless swelling of the scrotum that transilluminates. It often makes testicular palpation difficult and can conceal an underlying testicular tumor.

■ Congenital or Infant Hydroceles

Congenital or infant hydroceles are usually the result of peritoneal fluid accumulation within the scrotum via a patent processus vaginalis and occur in 6% of full-term boys. Their size often changes from day to day or with recumbency. Treatment should be delayed during the first year of life because normal spontaneous closure of the processus vaginalis may occur. After 1 year, surgical ligation of the processus vaginalis should be undertaken.

■ Acquired or Adult Hydroceles

Acquired or adult hydroceles are usually idiopathic but may be secondary to tumor, infection, or systemic disease. An imbalance in fluid secretion and absorption by the tunica vaginalis has been suggested as a possible cause. Treatment is generally indicated to allow easy palpation of the testis or because of symptomatic discomfort or disfigurement. Simple needle aspiration is an effective temporary treatment; however, the hydrocele will often recur. Injection of a sclerosing solution after aspiration can be successful in coapting the visceral and parietal layers of the tunica vaginalis and preventing reaccumulation of fluid. A mixture of 250 mg tetracycline diluted in 5 mL 0.5% bupivacaine (Marcaine) is often effective and minimizes the pain that accompanies injection. Sclerosing therapy is contraindicated with a patent processus vaginalis or an associated hernia. Definitive therapy is surgical drainage and excision of tunica vaginalis.

Spermatocele

A spermatocele is an epididymal retention cyst that arises from the efferent ductules and holds a cloudy fluid containing spermatozoa. It presents as a painless, cystic mass that lies above and anterior to the testis. Ultrasound can confirm the diagnosis if doubt exists. Treatment consists of spermatocelectomy and epididymectomy for extensive involvement. Aspiration or sclerosing therapy may result in epididymitis. Therapy should be avoided in young male patients concerned with fertility.

Varicocele

A varicocele is an abnormal dilatation of the veins of the pampiniform plexus and internal spermatic vein of the spermatic cord. Left-sided varicoceles are most common, occurring in approximately 15% of normal adult men. Unilateral right-sided varicoceles are rare (noted in only 2% of cases) and should suggest the possibility of compression or obstruction of the inferior vena cava (e.g., tumor or thrombus). Physical examination makes the diagnosis. Dilated veins are best palpated with the patient standing and aided by a Valsalva maneuver. Varicoceles have been described as feeling like a "bag of worms." The significance of a varicocele is its association with infertility. Indications for varicocelectomy include oligospermia, decreased sperm motility, and a painful symptomatic varicocele.

Trauma

Patients may have pain and swelling after blunt trauma to the scrotum. Differentiating a simple scrotal contusion from a fracture of the testicle can be difficult. Ultrasound can be helpful. Testicular fracture is almost always associated with a hematocele and should undergo surgical exploration. Simple contusions can be treated conservatively. Testicular torsion should always be suspected in the patient who has pain after minor scrotal trauma.

Paratesticular Tumors

Paratesticular tumors account for fewer than 10% of all intrascrotal tumors and can generally be differentiated from intratesticular masses by palpation and ultrasound. The adenomatoid tumor and lipoma of the cord are most common. Malignant tumors include rhabdomyosarcoma, fibrosarcoma, liposarcoma, and leiomyosarcoma.

Scrotal Edema

Lymphedema of the scrotum can present as markedly enlarged bilateral scrotal sacs. Potential causes include obstruction secondary to inflammation (filariasis, lymphogranuloma, tuberculosis, or syphilis), neoplasia, surgical procedures, or radiation.

DIAGNOSIS

The basic workup of a patient with scrotal pathology follows:
1. History
2. Physical examination with transillumination of the scrotum (use high-intensity light source if available)
3. Urinalysis
4. Color-flow Doppler ultrasound

The single most helpful piece of information is whether the patient has pain. A history of recent significant trauma also will narrow the diagnosis. Color-flow Doppler ultrasound is the best test to aid in the diagnosis of scrotal pathology.

■ Differential Diagnosis

Painful Scrotal Mass	Painless Scrotal Mass
Testicular torsion	Testicular tumor
Epididymitis	Hydrocele
Inguinal hernia	Inguinal hernia
Testicular tumor (rapidly growing)	Spermatocele
Trauma (testicular rupture)	Varicocele
	Paratesticular tumors

Pathology	Pain	Trans-illumination	Urinalysis	Ultrasound	Blood Flow
Testicular torsion	Yes	No	$\pm$	Solid	Negative
Testicular tumor	No	No	Negative	Solid	Normal
Testicular rupture	Yes	No	Negative	Complex	$\pm$
Epididymitis	Yes	No	Positive	Complex	Increased
Hydrocele	No	Yes	Negative	Cyst	Normal
Spermatocele	No	$\pm$	Negative	Cyst	Normal
Inguinal hernia	$\pm$	$\pm$	Negative	Complex	Normal

Empty Scrotum

Cryptorchidism is a common disorder in pediatric urology. It has been observed to occur in 3% of term infants and 30% of premature infants; however, 75% and 90% of these undescended testes, respectively, will have spontaneously descended by age 1 year, leaving a true incidence of close to 1% (0.8%) of the male population. Ten percent of cases are bilateral, 3% of which will have one or both testes absent. The etiology is unclear, and although many genetically inherited diseases have a high association with cryptorchidism, most cases of the undescended testis are isolated with no evidence of a genetic component.

SIGNIFICANCE

- A 20-fold increased risk of developing a testicular malignancy has been noted with undescended testes. Ten percent of testicular cancers arise in an undescended testis, 60% of which will be seminomas. The intraabdominal testis is four times more likely to undergo malignant degeneration than is an inguinal testis.
- Fertility is impaired. Only 30% of patients with bilateral cryptorchidism will be fertile. Spermatogenic damage appears to increase with higher position and longer periods of extrascrotal habitation.
- A high incidence of associated inguinal hernias (25%) occurs because of the patent processus vaginalis.
- An increased susceptibility to torsion exists, especially in the postpubertal period.

CLASSIFICATION

- *Intraabdominal (10%)*—testis is located proximal to the internal inguinal ring within the abdominal cavity.
- *Inguinal canal*—testis is located between internal and external inguinal rings.

- *Ectopic*—testis is located distal to the internal ring but outside its normal path of descent. Most are found in the superficial inguinal pouch or in the perineum, femoral canal, suprapubic area, and, rarely, in the contralateral scrotal compartment.
- *Absent testes (4%)*—20% of nonpalpable testes are absent.
- *Retractile testis*—testis is not truly undescended. Its extrascrotal location is secondary to hyperactive contraction of the cremasteric muscle. It is commonly found in the prescrotal or low inguinal area and with gentle manipulation can be placed in the scrotum without tension.

DIAGNOSIS

Carefully palpate both scrotal compartments, the inguinal canals, perineum, suprapubic area, and femoral canal. A *palpable testis* will be inguinal, ectopic, or retractile. If the testis can be easily placed within the scrotum without tension, it is retractile. Note that the cremasteric reflex is most active between ages 2 and 7 years, making this diagnosis difficult. A nonretractile palpable testis is either inguinal or ectopic.

A *nonpalpable testis* is either intraabdominal, ectopic, inguinal, or absent. If both testes are impalpable, then measure serum testosterone response to human chorionic gonadotropin (hCG) stimulation (hCG 2,000 IU qd × 3 days) and basal follicle-stimulating (FSH) and luteinizing hormone (LH) levels. A negative testosterone response to hCG and elevated basal FSH and LH levels are reliable evidence of anorchism (bilateral testicular absence). Bilateral or unilateral nonpalpable nondescensus can be further investigated by ultrasound, computed tomography, laparoscopy, and surgical exploration. Most testes will be found at surgery close to the internal inguinal ring.

TREATMENT

Why Treat Undescended Testis?

- To decrease the potential for malignant degeneration and to make the testis easier to palpate
- To improve prospects for fertility
- To repair inguinal hernias
- To decrease risk of torsion
- To avoid potential psychological complications

Therapy should be undertaken between ages 6 and 18 months. This will allow adequate time for spontaneous descent to occur and should minimize the potential complications of infertility and malignant degeneration. Retractile testes need no further therapy; however, periodic reexamination to confirm the diagnosis would be prudent. The truly undescended testes can be treated with either hormonal or surgical therapy or both.

Hormonal Therapy

Exogenous gonadotropin-releasing hormone or hCG has been reported to be successful in bringing down the testis in up to 70% and 50% of patients, respectively. Hormonal therapy is contraindicated with ectopic testes, in the setting of a hernia, and after prior orchiopexy or herniorrhaphy.

Surgical Therapy

Several different procedures for orchiopexy are effective, all based on the principles of adequate mobilization and fixation and repair of the associated hernia. Exploration for a nonpalpable testis is most commonly done with diagnostic laparoscopy. Orchiectomy should be performed if the testis cannot be placed in an easily palpable position and perhaps with all intraabdominal testes.

Urethral Discharge

PRESENTATION

Generally a young, sexually active male patient complains of ure-thral discharge (watery to purulent), with or without urethral burning or itching, and burning on urination. Urinary frequency and urgency are typically absent.

HISTORY

Ask about recent sexual contacts, history of venereal disease, and first onset of symptoms.

DIFFERENTIAL DIAGNOSIS

Gonococcal Urethritis

Gonococcal urethritis (GCU) has a short incubation of 1 to 5 days and generally produces a thick, purulent, yellowish discharge. The causative organism is *Neisseria gonorrhoeae*. Up to 30% of male patients with GCU also will be infected with *Chlamydia trachomatis*.

Nongonococcal Urethritis

Nongonococcal urethritis (NGU) has a long incubation of 5 to 21 days and generally produces a watery-to-mucoid, whitish discharge. The most common causative organisms include *C. trachomatis*, *Ureaplasma urealyticum*, *Trichomonas vaginalis*, and *Mycoplasma*.

WORKUP

Examination

Examination should be performed at least 1 hour after last void-ing and preferably 4 hours after voiding. (This is often a problem in the clinic setting because patients are generally instructed to give a urine specimen before seeing the doctor.) Notice whether the discharge is watery or thick, mucoid or purulent, and whitish or yellowish. Obtain a urethral specimen from within the urethra by using a calcium alginate (Calgiswab) urethrogenital swab for culture. (A drop of discharge is unacceptable.) Pharyngeal and rectal swabs also should be obtained if the history suggests exposure. Perform a routine genitourinary examination.

■ Culture Urethral Specimen

Culture on modified Thayer-Martin medium and New York City medium for *N. gonorrhoeae*. Suspicion of *C. trachomatis* requires culture on special media.

■ Gram's Stain of a Urethral Swab

The traditional Gram stain of a urethral swab specimen is generally not performed today, because modern antibiotic therapy will be directed against both GCU and NGU simultaneously. The presence of urethritis is confirmed by counting more than four polymorphonuclear leukocytes per oil immersion field ($\times 1,000$) from a Gram stain of a urethral swab. Demonstration of intracellular gram-negative diplococci within polymorphonuclear leukocytes is strong evidence of gonorrhea (99% specific and 95% sensitive in trained hands). No gram-negative cocci is strong evidence for NGU. Only extracellular gram-negative cocci are considered equivocal and nondiagnostic.

TREATMENT

Treatment should not await culture results because antibiotic therapy should cover both GCU and NGU. Azithromycin 2 g PO single dose is generally effective against both GCU and NGU. Ceftriaxone 125 mg IM once or cefixime 400 mg PO once or ciprofloxacin 500 mg PO or levofloxacin 250 mg single dose will effectively treat most GCU, although increasing resistance to fluoroquinolones has been noted in California, Hawaii, and Asia. The addition of doxycycline 100 mg PO bid $\times 7$ days will be effective against most NGU organisms. Every effort should be made to treat the patient's sexual partner (see Chapter 18).

Trauma

Traumatic injuries to the genitourinary tract represent about 10% of all injuries seen in the emergency room. The urgency of the patient's overall clinical condition will dictate how a diagnosis will be made. Care must be taken not to overlook significant urologic injuries during the commotion of a major trauma emergency. The initial assessment of major trauma will focus on control of hemorrhage and shock. Resuscitative efforts will usually require placement of intravenous (IV) lines and a Foley catheter. This early urologic intervention will be the first problem faced. Careful examination of the urethral meatus for the presence of blood is essential before Foley catheter placement. Blood at the meatus indicates urethral injury. A retrograde urethrogram can be performed to assess the extent of urethral injury before catheterization. The second urologic challenge will be to assess for renal injury in any major blunt abdominal trauma or penetrating trauma to the upper abdomen. This can be accomplished quickly by a double-dose (150 mL Renografin) bolus intravenous urogram (IVU) performed on the trauma table or, if possible, by computed tomography (CT) scan. Obtain urologic consultation before opening the abdomen.

INITIAL UROLOGIC ASSESSMENT

History

A detailed history of the traumatic event from the patient or eye-witnesses can help predict the type of injury.

Physical Examination

Injury to the bladder or urethra would be suggested by evidence of a pelvic fracture, blood at the urethral meatus, or superior displacement of the prostate on digital rectal examination. Diagnostic studies include
• Urinalysis

- Retrograde urethrogram if blood at the meatus
- CT scan with IV contrast
- Double-dose (150 mL) bolus IVU (for unstable patients)

RENAL INJURY

The kidney is the organ most commonly involved in urinary system trauma. Microscopic or gross hematuria indicates injury to the urinary system. However, 10% to 25% of significant renal injuries will present without hematuria, and these are most often major injuries of the renal pedicle. Renal injuries are properly separated into two major groups for diagnostic purposes: those caused by penetrating trauma (20%) and those caused by blunt trauma (80%).

Penetrating Renal Trauma

Penetrating trauma almost always results in surgical exploration because of other significant injuries (e.g., liver, small bowel, stomach, colon, and spleen). Gunshot and stab injuries are the most common causes. Renal injury can often be overlooked in the face of more urgent problems. Absence of hematuria does not rule out renal injury. A double-dose IVU can be performed on the operating table if no prior radiologic studies have been performed. CT scan with IV contrast should be obtained before going to the operating room if the patient's condition allows. Radiographic evidence of unilateral nonfunction, extravasation, suspected laceration, or large perirenal hematoma requires renal arteriography. Unfortunately, renal exploration of penetrating trauma often results in partial or total nephrectomy.

Blunt Renal Trauma

Blunt trauma requires considerable diagnostic effort to fully assess the extent of injury and determine proper management. Most blunt renal injuries result from rapid deceleration, as in a motor vehicle accident or a fall. Hematuria will usually be present, but its absence does not rule out renal injury. Patients with gross hematuria or microscopic hematuria [>5 red blood cells (RBCs) per high power field (hpf)] with shock should undergo imaging studies, usually a CT with IV contrast. Fracture of a lumbar transverse process or lower rib should raise suspicion of renal injury.

Classification of Renal Injury

Staging of renal trauma should begin with a double-dose (150 mL) IVU if the patient is hemodynamically unstable. This will effectively stage 85% of renal injuries. A CT scan with IV contrast is preferred if the patient is stable. Nonvisualization requires immediate renal arteriography without delay to evaluate for renal pedicle injury.

Minor Renal Trauma	Major Renal Trauma
Grade I—renal contusion or subcapsular hematoma	Grade III—cortical lacerations >1 cm without collecting system injury
Grade II—nonexpanding perirenal hematoma or laceration <1 cm	Grade IV—major lacerations of cortex; collecting system injury
	Grade V—renal pedicle injury; shattered kidney

Management of Blunt Renal Trauma

- Minor renal injury accounts for most cases and should be treated conservatively (bedrest until urine grossly clears, monitoring of vital signs and hematocrit).
- Renal pedicle injuries demand immediate surgery (revascularization or nephrectomy).
- Other major renal injuries can also be treated nonsurgically in most instances with careful monitoring, observation, and antibiotic coverage. Even grade IV lacerations can be cautiously monitored if the patient is stable and blood loss is limited.

Late Complications of Conservative Management

- Hypertension
- Abscess formation within urinoma or hematoma
- Delayed hemorrhage, which may occur 1 to 4 weeks after injury
- Hydronephrosis
- Arteriovenous fistula

URETERAL INJURY

Ureteral injury is usually the result of surgical mistakes resulting in ligation or transection; however, ureteral injury occasionally results from trauma, primarily gunshots. Hematuria will be present in 90% of traumatic ureteral injuries but in only 10% of surgical injuries. Diagnosis is made by demonstrating obstruction or extravasation on an excretory IVU with delayed films. A retrograde ureterogram can give precise preoperative localization. During a surgical procedure, suspicion of ureteral injury can be confirmed by giving 5 mL indigo carmine IV and inspecting for bluish extravasation. Delayed diagnosis is usually suggested by flank pain, abdominal tenderness, fever, paralytic ileus with nausea and vomiting, and occasionally ureterocutaneous or vaginal fistula.

Management of Ureteral Injury

- Immediately re-explore and repair with watertight tension-free anastomoses is the rule.
- Attempt to pass a retrograde or anterograde ureteral stent with incomplete or partial injuries.
- Options for *lower ureteral* injury:
  1. Antirefluxing reimplantation (first choice)
  2. Psoas hitch
  3. Boari bladder tube flap
- Options for *midureteral* injuries:
  1. Primary ureteroureterostomy
  2. Transureteroureterostomy (TUU)
- Options for *upper ureteral* injuries:
  1. Primary ureteroureterostomy
  2. Replacement with ileal segment
  3. Autotransplantation into pelvis
  4. Nephrectomy
- Stent with soft double-J ureteral catheters—generally recommended.
- Extraperitoneally drain all areas of possible extravasation.
- Antibiotic coverage should be given.

BLADDER INJURY

Bladder injury is caused by either penetrating trauma (usually gunshot) or blunt trauma (usually a motor vehicle accident). Blunt trauma resulting in lower urinary tract injury is usually the result of a pelvic fracture. Pelvic fractures have an associated lower urinary tract injury in about 15% of cases, with most involving the bladder. Fractures of the pubic rami are the most common type associated with lower urinary tract injury, with 20%

producing bladder injury. Blunt trauma can produce extraperitoneal perforations from bone fragments (80% of cases) and intraperitoneal rupture with a full bladder (20% of cases). Hematuria is present in almost 100%, with gross blood noted in more than 90%. Abdominal pain is also commonly noted.

Diagnosis of Bladder Injury

Diagnosis requires a distention cystogram with 300 to 400 mL dilute contrast and postdrainage films to detect small retrovesical extravasation. A false negative rate as high as 80% has been noted when less than 250 mL contrast is used. Excretory urography will only detect 15% of bladder injuries and is therefore an inadequate workup. A "teardrop" bladder deformity suggests a massive pelvic hematoma.

Management of Penetrating Bladder Injury

Prompt surgical exploration should be performed. Integrity of the lower ureters should be confirmed with 5 mL indigo carmine IV. Appearance of blue from the ureteral orifices should occur within 10 minutes. Suprapubic drainage should be provided by a large diameter (26–30 F) Malecot catheter and Penrose drains placed around the bladder. One should resist the temptation to explore a large pelvic hematoma.

Management of Blunt Bladder Injury

Intraperitoneal ruptures should be surgically explored with repair of the bladder injury. Placement of a suprapubic urinary catheter (24–30 F Malecot catheter) should be considered.

Extraperitoneal ruptures can be managed conservatively with simple Foley catheter drainage (20–22 F) and close monitoring in most instances. The catheter can generally be removed in 7 to 10 days but only after a satisfactory follow-up cystogram.

URETHRAL INJURY

Urethral injury is uncommon in males and even rarer in females. It typically results from either pelvic fractures or straddle type injuries. Anatomic localization to the posterior or anterior urethra aids in management.

Posterior Urethral Injuries

Posterior urethral injuries are usually the result of blunt trauma with a pelvic fracture, especially when involving the pubic rami. The primary site of injury is the prostatomembranous junction. The prostate is sheared from the membranous urethra that is anchored in the urogenital diaphragm. Patients present with blood at the meatus in more than 80% of cases, and digital rectal examination may reveal a high pelvic prostate. A retrograde urethrogram will demonstrate pelvic extraperitoneal extravasation above the urogenital diaphragm and usually also below. *Management* consists of suprapubic urinary diversion by open cystostomy with definitive repair in 3 to 6 months. Primary endoscopic realignment may be attempted if it can be accomplished easily and without disturbing the pelvic hematoma. An associated bladder rupture occurs in 20% of cases and should be repaired primarily without delay. *Complications* include stricture, impotence, and incontinence. Delayed primary repair of urethral injuries has been reported to decrease impotence and incontinence.

Anterior Urethral Injuries

Anterior urethral injuries are most often caused by a straddle fall or perineal trauma. Crushing of the bulbar urethra against the inferior margin of the symphysis pubis results in contusion or laceration. This type of injury accounts for less than 10% of all urethral injuries. Patients typically present with a bloody urethral discharge and a perineal bruise (butterfly hematoma). A retrograde urethrogram may demonstrate extravasation below the urogenital diaphragm. *Management* requires suprapubic drainage for 1 to 3 weeks if extravasation was noted. The catheter may be removed in 1 week if a voiding cystourethrography (VCUG) is normal. Occasionally, an extensive perineal hematoma with urinary extravasation will require primary surgical drainage. Stricture is the most common *complication*.

PENILE INJURIES

Penile injuries are usually the result of penetrating trauma from bullets or stab wounds or strangulation trauma from constricting rings. Fracture of the corpora cavernosa can occur from blunt trauma during a state of tumescence. The extent of injury is often readily apparent from physical examination. If Buck's fascia is intact, hematoma will be confined to the penis, whereas disruption of Buck's fascia will allow spread of the hematoma under Colles' and Scarpa's fascia onto the perineum and abdominal wall, respectively. A retrograde urethrogram and corpus cavernosography may be necessary to localize the injury.

Management of Penile Injuries

- *Avulsion of penile skin* distal to the injury should be removed and followed by a split-thickness skin graft.
- *Penetrating penile injury* deep to Colles' fascia should be explored.
- *Rupture of corpora cavernosa* is generally explored with evacuation of clots, debridement, and repair of the tunica albuginea.

SCROTAL AND TESTICULAR INJURY

Injuries to the scrotum are from either penetrating trauma (e.g., gunshot or stab wounds), blunt trauma, or burns. The severity of the injury will dictate the appropriate management; however, one should always suspect underlying testicular injury.

Penetrating Trauma

Management of scrotal lacerations must be guided by a thorough knowledge of the tissue layers involved.

Depth of Laceration	Management
Superficial (skin and dartos)	Primary debridement and closure
Deep to dartos	Surgical exploration
Tunica vaginalis entered	Penrose drain and primary closure
Through tunica albuginea	Necrotic or devitalized seminiferous tubules debrided and tunics closed primarily with absorbable suture

Blunt Scrotal Trauma

Whenever a history of minor scrotal trauma is given in the setting of swelling and pain, be sure to rule out testicular torsion or epididymitis. This can often be resolved by urinalysis. Pyuria suggests epididymitis. If torsion or testicular rupture is suspected, prompt exploration is recommended if any salvage is to be attained.

BURN INJURY

Burn injury to the genitalia requires careful monitoring because the extent of injury is often greater than is initially apparent. Management consists of debridement of devitalized tissue and topical therapy with silver sulfadiazine. A Foley catheter or suprapubic tube should be placed in extensively burned patients.

NEONATAL/PEDIATRIC

Abdominal Masses

More than 50% of neonatal abdominal masses arise from the kidney. Hydronephrosis and multicystic kidney are the most common etiologies, followed by polycystic kidney, renal vein thrombosis, and solid tumors. Workup should include careful physical examination and abdominal palpation, ultrasound, plain film, and intravenous (IV) urography. Note the immature neonatal kidney requires high doses of contrast, up to 4 mL/kg, because of its poor concentrating ability (see Chapter 15).

Hematuria

Hematuria in the neonate, particularly gross hematuria, is an emergency. Consider renal vein or artery thrombosis, renal cortical necrosis, obstructive uropathy, cystic renal disease, and tumors.

Hypertension

The kidney is the second most common cause of systemic hypertension in the neonate. Renal artery thrombosis is the most important etiology to rule out but also consider hydronephrosis secondary to obstruction or reflux, adrenogenital syndrome, and, rarely, pheochromocytoma, Cushing's disease, and hyperaldosteronism.

Delayed Micturition

Delay of micturition for more than 24 hours after birth, especially if associated with a distended palpable bladder, is cause for immediate concern. Ninety percent of newborns will have urinated about 10 mL within the first 24 hours of life. Consider lower urinary tract obstruction such as posterior urethral valves. Note that magnesium sulfate given to the mother for toxemia during delivery can cause transient neonatal urinary retention.

Scrotal Mass

A scrotal mass is rare in the neonate but must be given immediate attention. Consider torsion, epididymitis, incarcerated inguinal hernia, torsion of the appendix testis or epididymis, and testicular tumor. Management is generally surgical exploration (see Chapter 10).

Ambiguous Genitalia

Ambiguous genitalia are medical and social emergencies and require immediate evaluation (see Chapter 16).

Ascites

Urine is the most common reason for ascites in the neonate, and obstructive uropathy is the most common underlying cause. Posterior urethral valves and ureteropelvic junction obstruction are the most frequent etiologies, followed by urethral stricture or atresia, ectopic ureterocele, and neurogenic bladder. Voiding cystourethrography (VCUG) and IV urography are essential to diagnosis.

Renal Vein Thrombosis

Renal vein thrombosis can occur at any age but is most common in the neonatal period. Early diagnosis is dependent on having a high index of suspicion. Renal vein thrombosis in infancy equally affects males and females and left and right kidneys. More than half of the cases present within the first 2 weeks of life, most often in neonates with diarrhea and severe dehydration or in infants with diabetic mothers. Less commonly associated conditions include sepsis, traumatic deliveries, congenital heart disease, and maternal ingestion of thiazides or cytomegalovirus infection. Infants present with a flank mass, hematuria, thrombocytopenia, and nonvisualization of the involved kidney on IV urography.

Although once considered only for surgical therapy, unilateral renal vein thrombosis is now treated medically with correction of underlying disorders such as dehydration or sepsis.

Exstrophy

Cloacal exstrophy with its extensive array of problems will require immediate attention. Classic exstrophy should be considered for prompt surgical intervention within the first 24 to 48 hours in those patients who are suitable for reconstruction (see Chapter 34).

Absence of Abdominal Wall Musculature

Defective abdominal wall musculature should alert one to typical prune belly uropathy and may occasionally need prompt intervention (see Chapter 34).

Imperforate Anus

Imperforate anus, particularly with supralevator lesions, is associated with other urologic abnormalities in up to 50% of patients (see Chapter 34).

ADULT

Acute Urinary Retention

Acute urinary retention must be dealt with urgently to alleviate acute pain (see Chapter 1).

Testicular Torsion

Testicular torsion is less common in adults than in children. However, it must always head any list of differential diagnoses for an acute, painful testicular mass (see Chapter 10).

Priapism

The difficulty in treating and the complications arising from priapism increase significantly the longer the condition is allowed to exist. Early reversal is recommended (see Chapter 9).

Fournier's Gangrene

Fournier's gangrene is a rapidly fulminating, gangrenous infection of the genitalia. It begins as an extension of an infection from urinary, perianal, abdominal, or retroperitoneal sites or secondary to local trauma. A wide range of both aerobic and anaerobic organisms is encountered. It can present in any age group, but most occur after age 50. Most patients will have some underlying systemic disease, in particular diabetes. It often presents abruptly with severe pain of the penis, scrotum, or perineum, with rapid progression from erythema to necrosis, sometimes within hours. Other cases will have a more insidious onset with generalized symptoms of malaise, fever, chills or sweats, and genital discomfort. A mortality rate of up to 50% has been reported.

■ Diagnosis

A careful history should be taken with special attention to possible underlying disorders such as diabetes mellitus, immunosuppression, steroid medications, alcohol abuse, or other infections. The physical diagnosis is not difficult. Areas of erythema, induration, skin necrosis, and crepitus are usual, and the overwhelming fetid odor is unmistakable. It is important to determine the full extent of the process and to search for the source, particularly in the anorectal and urogenital areas. The infection not uncommonly extends all the way up the abdominal wall. Proctoscopy and a retrograde urethrogram may be helpful.

■ Management

The mainstay of treatment is aggressive surgical debridement and triple drug antibiotic therapy. Blood, urine, and wound cultures should be taken before starting antibiotic therapy. Metronidazole (Flagyl), ampicillin, and gentamicin are reasonable choices for initial therapy. Immediate surgical debridement under anesthesia must follow. An exploratory laparotomy or diverting colostomy is occasionally necessary. After debridement, the wounds are left open and packed with fine-mesh gauze soaked in Dakin's solution (hypochlorite—Clorox). Dressings should be changed two to three times a day. Antibiotics should be continued until there is no evidence of active infection and the wound is clean with a base of granulation tissue.

Autonomic Dysreflexia

Autonomic dysreflexia is a syndrome characterized by a major sympathetic nervous response to afferent visceral stimulation in the patient with spinal cord injury. Clinical manifestations include dangerous systolic hypertension, sweating, a pounding headache, paradoxical bradycardia, a widened pulse pressure, and a subjective sense of impending doom on the part of the patient. This can occur in response to stimulation of the bladder, urethra, or rectum in patients with cord lesions above T6, usually in the cervical region, and most frequently during the 3 to 8 months after injury. Acute bladder filling as occurs during cystoscopy or urodynamic testing can trigger an episode. Catheter drainage of the bladder can be used to minimize chronic autonomic dysreflexia.

■ Treatment

In a hypertensive crisis, sodium nitroprusside (50 mg in 250 mL of D5W) can be titrated IV to bring pressure down within 5 minutes (1–3 µg/kg per minute). An α-blocker such as phentolamine (Regitine) 5 mg IV bolus can also be used to treat an acute episode along with removal of the afferent stimulus (i.e., drain the bladder). Chlorpromazine (Thorazine), 25 mg intramuscular (IM) every 6 hours (q6h), and oral α-blockers can be used prophylactically in patients with the potential for such a response during cystoscopy. Spinal anesthesia will block dysreflexia during surgery better than a general anesthetic.

Lower Extremity Weakness in Advanced Prostate Cancer

Occasionally, patients present with untreated metastatic prostate cancer and signs of incipient spinal cord compression (e.g., lower extremity weakness and lax anal sphincter tone). These patients need emergency treatment to decrease tumor mass and relieve the cord compression. Motor function is lost first with spinal cord compression, and pinprick sensation is the last to go. Patients who have retained pinprick sensation may safely be given a trial of other forms of treatment before resorting to a decompression laminectomy. Neurologic consultation should be obtained. Options for treatment are as follows:
- Emergency bilateral orchiectomies
- Ketoconazole [400 mg orally (PO) every 8 hours (q8h)]
- IV diethylstilbestrol (Stilphostrol)
- Radiotherapy
- Emergency decompression laminectomy

Abdominal Masses

PEDIATRICS

An abdominal mass in children most commonly arises from the urinary tract or adrenals and should therefore be worked up by a urologist until imaging studies prove otherwise. A hydronephrotic kidney secondary to ureteropelvic junction (UPJ) obstruction is the most common cause of a unilateral abdominal mass in childhood, followed by a multicystic kidney. Neuroblastomas or Wilms' tumors are the most common causes of a solid abdominal mass in children.

■ Differential Diagnosis of Abdominal Mass in Children

Cystic Lesions	Solid Lesions
Hydronephrosis—ureteropelvic junction obstruction	Neuroblastoma
Multicystic kidney	Wilms' tumor
Adrenal hemorrhage	Mesoblastic nephroma
Ovarian cyst	Hepatoblastoma
Intestinal duplication anomaly	
Mesenteric cyst	

Imaging Techniques

1. Ultrasound should be the first imaging study performed. It will provide differentiation of solid from fluid- or blood-filled masses in most cases and give localization to a specific area of the abdomen.
2. Intravenous (IV) urography is often unsatisfactory during the first weeks of life because of the poor concentrating ability of the neonatal kidney. However, it provides valuable anatomic and functional detail for diagnosis of retroperitoneal masses. The addition of a furosemide (Lasix) washout test can help identify partial obstruction.
3. Mertiatide (MAG3) renal scan with Lasix is an alternative first choice for the clearly cystic mass. It will give information on renal function and identify partial UPJ obstruction.

4. Computed tomography (CT) will give more accurate anatomic localization of solid masses and help further differentiate equivocal masses as solid versus cystic.
5. Voiding cystourethrography (VCUG) should be performed on all hydronephrotic masses to differentiate obstruction from reflux.
6. Anterograde pyelography via a percutaneous nephrostomy is often helpful to determine the level of obstruction while providing urinary drainage and information on the potential for functional recovery of the kidney.
7. Cystoscopy with retrograde pyelography will provide information on the status of the lower ureter and bladder when needed.

ADULTS

Renal masses are increasingly being discovered incidentally during abdominal CT scans, ultrasound, or IV urography performed for unrelated reasons. These masses will require further workup for definitive diagnosis and treatment if indicated. The classic triad of flank mass, flank pain, and hematuria that heralds a renal cell carcinoma occurs in only less than 10% of patients.

■ Differential Diagnosis of a Flank Mass in Adults

Cystic Lesions	Solid Lesions
Renal tumors	Renal tumors
Simple renal cyst	Renal cell carcinoma
Complex renal cyst	Angiomyolipoma
Hydronephrosis	Renal oncocytoma
Multicystic kidney	Pseudotumor
Renal abscess	Hemangiopericytoma
Adult polycystic kidney	Renal sarcoma
	Transitional cell carcinoma
	Xanthogranulomatous pyelonephritis
Adrenal tumors	Adrenal tumors
Adrenal cyst	Adrenal carcinoma
	Adrenal adenoma
	Pheochromocytoma
	Metastatic tumor

Imaging Techniques (see Chapter 36)

• Ultrasound is the simplest method of differentiating a solid from cystic structure, and a cyst can be diagnosed with 98% accuracy if all criteria are met.

- IV urography is still the best imaging technique for the renal collecting system and gives good definition of a renal mass when tomography is used. Improved diagnostic and staging accuracy can be obtained from CT or magnetic resonance imaging (MRI).
- CT scan first without and then with IV contrast enhancement is the single best method to evaluate a retroperitoneal flank mass. It discriminates well between solid and cystic lesions and can often demonstrate renal vein and/or inferior vena caval extension.
- MRI is an important modality for evaluating abdominal mass. Renal vein and inferior vena cava extension can be accurately determined. MRI can be used in patients who cannot receive IV contrast agents because of contrast allergy, renal insufficiency, or renal failure. MRI with gadolinium-diethylenetriamine pentaacetic acid (DTPA) has no nephrotoxic effects.
- Cyst puncture by ultrasound or CT guidance for cysts that do not meet the full criteria of a simple cyst may be helpful.
- Renal arteriography can demonstrate the classic hypervascularity of renal cell carcinoma; however, it has largely been displaced by CT scans and MRI for diagnostic purposes. Arteriography is still indicated when vascular anatomy is needed to help plan a partial nephrectomy.
- Venacavography should be performed if renal vein and inferior vena cava involvement is in doubt.

Renal Cysts

Approximately 20% to 25% of routine ultrasonography and abdominal CT scans reveal unexpected renal cysts. Differentiating simple cysts (benign) from complex renal cysts (15% potentially malignant) can be a challenge. Using the Bosniak classification can help categorize various renal cysts to help make clinical management decisions. Renal ultrasound and a renal protocol CT scan (thin section without and with IV contrast) are the most useful diagnostic techniques. Differentiation of Bosniak II and III cysts can be difficult.

■ Bosniak I—Simple Cyst

A simple renal cyst has thin walls, no internal echoes or septations, no calcifications, and CT Hounsfield units (HU) of 0 to 20 with no contrast enhancement. These are extremely common and require no further workup.

■ Bosniak II—Benign Minimally Complex Cyst

Bosniak II cysts can include a few thin septa, minimal calcification, infected cysts, and high-density hemorrhagic cysts. These have low malignant potential and can be treated nonsurgically. If any criteria are in question, then these cysts should be followed with repeat CT scan in 3 to 6 months and annually as indicated.

■ Bosniak III—Moderately Complex Cyst

These are truly indeterminate cysts, with 50% of these lesions being malignant. Bosniak III cysts have numerous or thick septa, thickened walls, irregular calcification, or multiloculated features. These cysts should generally be managed with surgical exploration and partial nephrectomy if technically feasible.

■ Bosniak IV—Cystic Malignant Tumors

These are characterized by enhancing nodular walls or obvious solid components. Greater than 90% of these will prove to be malignant and should be managed with partial or radical nephrectomy.

Hydronephrosis

Hydronephrosis can be detected by ultrasound and is best evaluated by IV urography and retrograde studies.

Solid Tumor

A solid tumor by ultrasound can best be localized to the kidney or adrenal by CT or MRI. A solitary solid renal tumor must be presumed to be renal cell carcinoma and should undergo surgical removal (see Chapter 24). An exception is a solid renal tumor with clear evidence of fat within the tumor on CT scan (-50 to -150 HU). This is strong evidence for an angiomyolipoma and may be followed up. An adrenal tumor will require the appropriate workup (see Chapter 25).

Tumor Calcifications

Calcifications, although occurring in less than 5% of renal masses, increase the suspicion of malignancy. Mottled central calcifications indicate a solid mass and are usually a sign of renal cell carcinoma (>90% specificity). A peripheral calcification, although often a cyst, is associated with renal cell carcinoma in at least 20% of cases.

Cystic Lesions	Solid Lesions
Hydronephrosis–ureteropelvic junction obstruction	Neuroblastoma
Multicystic kidney	Wilms' tumor
Adrenal hemorrhage	Mesoblastic nephroma
Ovarian cyst	Hepatoblastoma
Intestinal duplication anomaly	
Mesenteric cyst	
Renal tumors	Renal tumors
Simple renal cyst	Renal cell carcinoma
Complex renal cyst	Angiomyolipoma
Hydronephrosis	Renal oncocytoma
Multicystic kidney	Pseudotumor
Renal abscess	Hemangiopericytoma
Adult polycystic kidney	Renal sarcoma
	Transitional cell carcinoma
	Xanthogranulomatous
	pyelonephritis
Adrenal tumors	Adrenal tumors
Adrenal cyst	Adrenal carcinoma
	Adrenal adenoma
	Pheochromocytoma
	Metastatic tumor

16 Ambiguous Genitalia

Evaluation of the newborn with ambiguous genitalia is a medical and social emergency. Early sex assignment will help to resolve the social implications for the family. No other decision will have such a profound impact on the child and family. A clear understanding of the pathophysiology is essential if a correct decision is to be made expeditiously.

MECHANISMS OF SEXUAL DIFFERENTIATION

The process of normal sexual differentiation is a series of staged modifications of bilateral tissue primordia. However, these modifications appear to be controlled by local factors, independent from one side to the other.

Development of Gonads

The genetic sex is determined at the time of fertilization by the delivery of an X or Y chromosome by the sperm. The normal female is 46XX and the normal male is 46XY. The medullary portion of the indifferent gonad develops into a testis under the influence of the protein product of the SRY (sex-determining region of the Y chromosome) gene, a product of the short arm of the Y chromosome, also known as the testis determining factor (TDF). In the absence of the SRY protein, the cortex of the indifferent gonad develops into an ovary by default. By the seventh week of gestation the gonadal sex has been established.

Development of Internal Ducts

By the sixth week of gestation, two paired internal duct systems derived from the mesonephric renal system exist side by side. The mesonephric (wolffian) duct will give rise to male structures, and the paramesonephric (müllerian) duct will become female structures. Male differentiation is dependent on testicular production of müllerian-inhibitory substance (MIS) from fetal Sertoli's cells and testosterone secretion by fetal Leydig's cells. Following regression of the müllerian duct under the influence of MIS, the wolffian duct will develop into the epididymis, vas deferens, and seminal vesicles under the influence of testosterone. In the absence of MIS and testosterone, the müllerian duct will evolve into the fallopian tubes, uterus, and upper third of the vagina, and the wolffian duct will passively degenerate.

Development of External Genitalia

The external genitalia develop from the urogenital sinus, genital tubercle, genital folds, and genital swellings. Male development is dependent on the ability of these tissues to convert testosterone into dihydrotestosterone by the enzyme 5-α-reductase. Female differentiation is essentially the unmodified embryologic state that persists in the absence of these hormones.

Tissue Primordia	Female (Unmodified Differentiation)	Male (Requires 5-α-reductase)
Urogenital sinus	Lower vagina and Skene's duct	Prostate
Genital tubercle	Clitoris	Glans penis
Genital folds	Labia minora	Urethra and shaft of penis
Genital swellings	Labia majora	Scrotum

DISORDERS OF SEXUAL DIFFERENTIATION

Not all disorders of intersexuality produce ambiguous genitalia. Numerous distinct disorders of chromosomal, gonadal, or phenotypic development have been described. Patients may present with infertility, delayed puberty, or primary amenorrhea. All disorders of ambiguous genitalia are the result of abnormal virilization (e.g., virilization of a genetic female, incomplete virilization of a genetic male, or partial virilization because of defective genetic assignment). Only those disorders that commonly present with ambiguous genitalia in the newborn are reviewed.

Female Pseudohermaphroditism

The female pseudohermaphrodite is an example of virilization of a 46XX genetic female with normal ovaries secondary to excessive endogenous or exogenous intrauterine androgens. It is the most frequent etiology for ambiguous genitalia, and congenital adrenal hyperplasia is the most common reason for virilization.

- Congenital adrenal hyperplasia occurs secondary to a defect in the glucocorticoid synthesis pathway (see figure on p. 176), resulting in decreased cortisol production and positive feedback on the anterior pituitary to increase adrenocorticotropic hormone (ACTH) release. Elevated ACTH levels cause adrenal hyperplasia and increased adrenal androgen synthesis. A defect in 21-hydroxylase with salt-losing symptoms accounts for about 90% of cases. The remaining 10% are due to a deficiency of 11-β-hydroxylase with associated salt retention.
- Other causes of excessive androgens include exogenous maternal ingestion of certain progestins or maternal virilizing tumors such as arrhenoblastomas or luteomas.

Mixed Gonadal Dysgenesis

Mixed gonadal dysgenesis is an abnormality of sex chromosome number, with the most common karyotype being 46XY/45X0 mosaic. Most patients are poorly virilized and infertile, so most are raised as females. Mixed gonadal dysgenesis is reported to be the second most frequent cause of ambiguous genitalia; 25% of patients will develop testicular gonadoblastomas if reared as males.

Male Pseudohermaphroditism

The male pseudohermaphrodite is an example of an incompletely virilized 46XY genetic male with normal testes. Causes include defective androgen synthesis, defective androgen action, deficient 5-α-reductase activity (pseudovaginal perineoscrotal hypospadias), or deficient MIS (hernia uteri inguinale). When the androgen defect is severe, patients may have completely feminine external genitalia with intraabdominal testes (complete testicular feminization).

True Hermaphroditism

The true hermaphrodite is rare. These individuals have both testicular and ovarian elements; a uterus is usually present, as are internal ducts that correspond to the gonad on that side (e.g., testis, ovary, or ovotestis). The most common karyotype is 46XX (80%). Differentiation of the external genitalia is variable, and hypospadias is common.

WORKUP

History

Take a detailed family history of any abnormal sexual development, including unexplained fetal deaths, infertility, amenorrhea, and hirsutism. Question the mother about any medications or drugs taken during pregnancy (e.g., progestational agents are converted to androgens).

Physical Examination

Examine the infant carefully for a palpable gonad in the labioscrotal fold or scrotum that would exclude the diagnosis of female pseudohermaphroditism. Hyperpigmentation of the areola or labioscrotal folds suggests elevated levels of ACTH (ACTH shares a common subunit with melanocyte-stimulating hormone) and therefore congenital adrenal hyperplasia. Evidence of dehydration suggests a salt-losing (21-hydroxylase deficiency) congenital adrenal hyperplasia, whereas significant hypertension suggests sodium retention (11-β-hydroxylase deficiency). Attempt to palpate a uterus in the lower abdomen. Document the size of the phallus and the position of the urethral meatus.

Biochemical Studies

▪ **Plasma Measurements**

- 17-OH-progesterone elevation after the first 36 hours of life suggests 21-hydroxylase deficiency (upper limit of normal 200 ng/dL).
- 11-Deoxycortisol elevation suggests 11-β-hydroxylase deficiency.
- Testosterone levels before and after human chorionic gonadotropin (hCG) stimulation (2,000 IU/day for 4 days) in the male pseudohermaphrodite are helpful in differentiating androgen resistance from a defect in androgen synthesis.

- Testosterone and dihydrotestosterone levels are helpful in identifying 5-α-reductase deficiency and androgen insensitivity syndromes.
- Serum electrolytes should be obtained.

■ Urinary Measurements

- 17-Ketosteroids are metabolites of adrenal androgens (normal <15 mg/24 hours).
- Pregnanetriol is a metabolite of 17-OH-progesterone.

■ Cultured Skin Fibroblasts

Cultured skin fibroblasts can be used to test for androgen resistance when necessary.

Special Studies

Genitography can be performed by injecting contrast into the urogenital sinus under fluoroscopic control.

Endoscopy can define the presence of a cervix and help perform genitography.

Ultrasonography can help document the presence of a uterus and fallopian tubes and thereby rule out male pseudohermaphroditism.

Exploratory laparotomy or laparoscopy and gonadal biopsy may become necessary.

Chromosome Studies

■ Buccal Smear

The presence of a Barr body (chromatin clumps on the nuclear membrane) within cells from the buccal mucosa can quickly suggest the genetic sex. The Barr body, which represents the second X chromosome, is found in more than 20% of the cells of a normal female and less than 2% of the cells of a normal male.

■ Karyotype Analysis

Karyotype analysis should be performed from cultured peripheral blood leukocytes arrested in metaphase. This will provide detailed chromosomal information; however, the results are usually not available for 3 to 4 days.

Sex Assignment

No other medical intervention will have such a profound effect on the life of the patient. Sex assignment should be made with family consultation and only after all studies are complete. Every attempt should be made to rear children based on their genetic assignment.

Genital Reconstruction

Appropriate reconstruction of the external genitalia is best delayed until after some time for normal growth is allowed. Reconstruction between age 6 and 12 months is reasonable.

Part Two

Selected Topics

17 Urinary Tract Infections

Urinary tract infections (UTIs) are common and potentially disabling. It is important to use the same terminology when referring to various types of infectious episodes. Bacteriuria is merely the presence of bacteria in the urine, whereas a UTI implies an inflammatory response to bacterial invasion of the tissues. Pyuria is the presence of white blood cells (WBCs) in the urine seen on microscopic urinalysis and is an indication of an inflammatory process.

CLASSIFICATION OF URINARY TRACT INFECTIONS

1. First infection
2. Unresolved bacteriuria during therapy (most commonly owing to a resistant organism)
3. Recurrent UTIs:
   a. *Reinfection (>80%)*—recurrence from new organisms outside the urinary tract
   b. *Bacterial persistence (uncommon)*—recurrence from the same organism within the urinary tract despite sterilization of urine during therapy

Causes of Bacterial Persistence

- Infected stones
- Chronic bacterial prostatitis
- Unilateral infected atrophic kidney
- Vesicovaginal or intestinal fistulas
- Ureteral anomalies
- Infected diverticula
- Foreign bodies (stents, catheters)
- Infected urachal cyst
- Infected medullary sponge kidney
- Infected papillary necrosis
- Ureteral stump after nephrectomy

Factors That Increase Risk of Complications from Urinary Tract Infections

- Urinary tract obstruction
- Infections from urea-splitting bacteria
- Diabetes mellitus
- Renal papillary necrosis
- Neurogenic bladders
- Pregnancy
- Congenital urinary tract anomalies
- Elderly patient with acute bacterial prostatitis
- Severe reflux in children younger than 4 years
- End-stage renal disease on hemodialysis
- Immunosuppression after a renal transplant

UPPER TRACT INFECTIONS

Acute Pyelonephritis

Acute pyelonephritis is associated with a clinical syndrome of chills, fever, and flank pain as a result of bacterial infection of the renal parenchyma and pelvis. It is usually associated with dysuria, pyuria, frequency, and urgency. The most common causative organisms are *Escherichia coli*, *Klebsiella*, *Proteus*, *Enterobacter*, *Pseudomonas*, *Serratia*, *Citrobacter*, occasionally *Streptococcus fecalis*, and rarely *Staphylococcus aureus*. Infection usually results from bacteria ascending from the lower urinary tract. Hematogenous infection occurs infrequently.

■ Workup

1. Urinalysis (pyuria, bacteriuria, hematuria)
2. Urine culture and sensitivity (before and during therapy)
3. Complete blood count (CBC) (significant neutrophilic leukocytosis)
4. Blood culture (frequently positive)
5. Noncontrast CT of abdomen and pelvis or intravenous urography (IVU) (may show stones or obstruction)
6. Renal ultrasound (stones, hydronephrosis, or abscess)
7. Voiding cystourethrography (VCUG) (delay several weeks because transient reflux can often occur during an acute infection)

■ Differential Diagnosis

Differential diagnosis includes pancreatitis, basal pneumonia, appendicitis, cholecystitis, diverticulitis, and pelvic inflammatory disease.

■ Management

In uncomplicated cases, outpatient management with an oral fluoroquinolone may be appropriate. In others, intravenous (IV) antibiotic therapy should be started without delay after cultures are sent. A quinolone or ampicillin [1 g IV every 6 hours (q6h)] and gentamicin or tobramycin [1.5 mg/kg IV every 8 hours (q8h)] are a good choice initially until culture and sensitivity results are available. Obstruction noted on imaging studies must be relieved. Fevers will often persist for 2 to 5 days despite sterile urine and antibiotic therapy. However, if the urine continues to show infection, reevaluation should be instituted to rule out obstruction, abscess, or inappropriate antibiotic selection. If symptoms have resolved after 2 to 5 days of IV antibiotics, the patient may be switched to oral (PO) medication for an additional 10 to 14 days.

Pyonephrosis

Pyonephrosis refers to a patient with acute pyelonephritis complicated by obstructed hydronephrosis. The IVU will show nonfunction or poor visualization of the involved kidney. Renal ultrasound or CT scan can usually make the diagnosis. Fifty percent of obstructed pyonephrotic kidneys are nonfunctioning. Obstruction should always be ruled out in pyelonephritis. Renal ultrasound is usually sufficient.

■ Management

IV antibiotics and immediate relief of obstruction by either a percutaneous nephrostomy or placement of a retrograde ureteral stent are mandatory.

Emphysematous Pyelonephritis

Emphysematous pyelonephritis is an acute necrotizing parenchymal and perirenal infection. It is a rare complication of acute pyelonephritis in which organisms (generally *E. coli*) ferment glucose to CO_2 and H_2O, producing gas in the renal parenchyma. The characteristic appearance of intraparenchymal gas on kidney, ureter, and bladder (KUB) study is diagnostic. Eighty percent of cases occur in poorly controlled insulin-dependent diabetics, and the rest occur in patients with obstruction. Prognosis is poor with a high mortality.

Management consists of IV antibiotics, relief of obstruction, and frequently nephrectomy.

Renal Abscess (Carbuncle)

Renal cortical or medullary abscesses typically arise from a focus of pyelonephritis (usually *E. coli*) or by hematogenous spread of *S. aureus* from a distant cutaneous infection, particularly in IV drug abusers. Patients present with chills, fever, and flank pain. Urinalysis may be normal in a staphylococcal renal abscess. CBC will show marked leukocytosis with a shift to the left.

▪ Diagnosis

Renal ultrasound or computed tomography (CT) scan can usually make the diagnosis. Percutaneous needle aspiration of the mass will confirm the diagnosis.

▪ Treatment

Initial therapy should be IV antibiotics. Staphylococcal abscesses should be treated with a β-lactamase-resistant penicillin such as nafcillin. Ampicillin and gentamicin or third-generation cephalosporins are appropriate for a gram-negative abscess. Drainage by percutaneous aspiration or surgical incision may be necessary. Nephrectomy is rarely needed.

Perinephric Abscess

A perinephric abscess lies between the renal capsule and the perirenal (Gerota's) fascia. Rupture of an intrarenal abscess into the perirenal space is the most common etiology; however, hematogenous seeding from distant sites of infection occurs. The most common organisms are *Proteus* or *E. coli* (from an intrarenal abscess) and *S. aureus* (from distant infections). Mortality has been reported to be as high as 50%, mostly because of the difficulty in making a diagnosis. Diabetics and patients with polycystic kidneys on hemodialysis are particularly susceptible.

▪ Diagnosis

Diagnosis is best made by renal ultrasound and CT scan aided by diagnostic needle aspiration.

Treatment

The primary treatment of a perinephric abscess is percutaneous or surgical drainage. Antibiotics are needed to control sepsis. Nephrectomy may be indicated if the kidney is nonfunctioning or severely infected.

Chronic Pyelonephritis

Chronic pyelonephritis is a radiologic (IVU) or pathologic diagnosis referring to severe cortical scarring or the small, contracted, atrophic kidney. Etiology is unclear; however, chronic pyelonephritis appears to originate in childhood and is associated with recurrent bacteriuria and vesicoureteral reflux.

Xanthogranulomatous Pyelonephritis

Xanthogranulomatous pyelonephritis is an uncommon, atypical chronic renal parenchymal infection that is often misdiagnosed as a renal tumor. Etiology is unknown, but infection and obstruction are almost always present.

Presentation

Fever, chills, flank pain, and flank mass are typical. The IVU shows a renal mass in 60% and stones in 40% to 70%. CT scan often demonstrates a large renal mass with a central calcification. The involved kidney is often nonfunctioning. Persistent bacteriuria occurs in less than 50%, with *Proteus* and *E. coli* being the most frequent organisms. It can be difficult to differentiate from renal cell carcinoma; therefore, the diagnosis is often made at surgical exploration.

Treatment

Partial or total nephrectomy is the usual treatment.

LOWER TRACT INFECTIONS

Cystitis

Acute bacterial cystitis is an infection of the bladder with organisms that ascended from the urethra. Its hallmark symptoms include frequency, urgency, nocturia, and dysuria. Patients will often complain of low back or suprapubic pain. Fever is unusual.

Urinalysis typically shows pyuria, bacteriuria, and hematuria. Urine cultures are positive, and *E. coli* is the usual pathogen. A persistent *Proteus* infection should suggest the possibility of an infected struvite stone.

Females have a higher incidence of cystitis, which increases throughout their lifetime. Recurrence is also high and is associated with coliform bacterial colonization of the urethra and vaginal vestibule.

Males are more likely to have other associated urinary problems (e.g., prostatitis, urethritis, strictures, or benign prostatic hyperplasia) that must be treated.

Children with a UTI, particularly infants, should have a thorough evaluation of the urinary tract, including VCUG and renal ultrasound. (VCUG should be postponed 4 to 6 weeks because incidental low-grade reflux is often observed during an acute infection.)

■ Treatment

Short course (3 days) or single-dose therapy has been shown to be as effective as 7 to 14 days of therapy in adult nondiabetic females and children with uncomplicated lower UTIs of less than 2 days' duration. Sulfonamides, trimethoprim-sulfamethoxazole (TMP-SMX), and nitrofurantoins are usually effective agents for initial therapy. Antibiotic choice should always be guided by sensitivity testing when available.

Pyocystitis

Pyocystitis is a collection of pus within the bladder. It most commonly occurs in dialysis patients with low or absent urine output. Patients present with fever, suprapubic pain, and a palpable mass. Pelvic ultrasound can help make the diagnosis; however, a strong suspicion would warrant a diagnostic bladder aspiration. Management involves draining the bladder and providing appropriate antibiotic coverage.

Emphysematous Cystitis

Emphysematous cystitis (cystitis emphysematosa) is a rare manifestation of UTI characterized by gas within the bladder or its muscular wall. It usually occurs in severe diabetics and is commonly caused by *E. coli*, *Proteus*, *Pseudomonas*, and rarely *Clostridia*. Certain strains of these bacteria have the potential to ferment glucose. Other causes of air in the bladder include instrumentation and colovesical fistulas. The radiographic picture on KUB is pathognomonic. Cystography will confirm the location of the gas in the bladder. Treatment includes appropriate antibiotic therapy, control of glucosuria, and relief of any outlet obstruction.

Urethritis in Males

Urethritis in males presents with urethral discharge, dysuria, and frequency. It is an infection acquired by inoculation of organisms into the urethra during sexual intercourse. It is classified as gonococcal or nongonococcal urethritis based on the causative pathogens.

■ Gonococcal Urethritis

Gonococcal urethritis is caused by an intracellular gram-negative diplococcus, *Neisseria gonorrhoeae*. It has a short incubation of 2 to 8 days and produces a purulent, yellowish discharge with dysuria.

Diagnosis

Diagnosis is based on a history of sexual contact, a purulent discharge with dysuria, and a positive Gram stain and/or culture. The specimen for culture and the Gram stain must be carefully taken from within the urethra using a calcium alginate (Calgiswab) urethrogenital swab at least 1 hour after the patient last voided. A modified Thayer-Martin culture medium should be directly inoculated.

Treatment

Treatment should not await culture results even if the Gram stain is negative when suspicion is high. Appropriate regimens would include ceftriaxone 125 mg intramuscularly (IM), ciprofloxacin 500 mg PO, or ofloxacin 400 mg PO. *Chlamydia* coverage is also achieved with azithromycin 1.0 g PO or doxycycline 100 mg PO bid for 7 days.

■ Nongonococcal Urethritis

Nongonococcal urethritis is believed to be the most common cause of urethritis in males, with *Chlamydia trachomatis* being the most important pathogen (40%). Other likely pathogens include *Ureaplasma urealyticum* (30%), *Trichomonas vaginalis* (5%), and *Candida albicans*. It has a prolonged incubation of 5 to 21 days and produces a mucoid, whitish discharge, with or without dysuria. The diagnosis of nongonococcal urethritis requires the exclusion of gonorrhea and the demonstration of urethritis (a Gram stain of urethral swab showing >4 polymorphonucleocytes per oil immersion field).

Treatment

Azithromycin 1 g PO in a single dose, doxycycline 100 mg PO twice a day (bid) for 7 days, or ofloxacin (Floxin) 300 mg PO bid for 7 days is appropriate for *Chlamydia* or *Ureaplasma*. If *T. vaginalis* is suspected, then metronidazole 2 g PO single dose or 250 mg PO three times a day (tid) for 7 days should be given.

▪ Reiter's Syndrome

Reiter's syndrome is a rare complication of nongonococcal urethritis possibly owing to *C. trachomatis*. It can present with arthritis, conjunctivitis, balanitis circinata, or keratodermia blennorrhagia.

Urethritis in Females

Urethritis in females presents with frequency, dysuria, and often pyuria; however, the urine culture will show no growth. Vaginitis accounts for up to one third of these cases and must be diagnosed and treated appropriately. Gonorrhea or chlamydial infection will be responsible for urethritis in most other patients, despite the absence of a urethral discharge, and is treated as done so in males.

Vaginitis

Vaginitis often produces symptoms that mimic a bladder infection and, therefore, must be recognized so that appropriate treatment may be rendered. Normal vaginal discharge is clear, white, or gray, with a pH of less than 4.5, and rare leukocytes. The most common causes of adult vaginitis are *Trichomonas*, *Candida*, and nonspecific organisms.

▪ *Trichomonas* Vaginitis

Trichomonas vaginitis is caused by a flagellated protozoan, *T. vaginalis*, and produces a thin, watery, yellowish-green, foamy malodorous discharge. Patients present with soreness, itching, and dysuria. The discharge may liberate a fishy odor with 10% potassium hydroxide (KOH), has a pH of greater than 4.5, and will show leukocytes and motile trichomonads. *Trichomonas* culture is positive.

Treatment

Use one dose of metronidazole (Flagyl) 2 g PO or 500 mg PO bid for 7 days. (Note: patients should abstain from drinking alcohol while on Flagyl.) In pregnancy, clotrimazole vaginal suppositories should be used.

■ Candida Vaginitis

Candida vaginitis (*Monilia*) is generally caused by C. *albicans* and produces a thick, white, cheesy, curd-like discharge. Mycotic or fungal vaginitis most often occurs in pregnancy and diabetes and in patients taking oral contraceptives or antibiotics, especially tetracycline. Patients present with intense itching and discharge that shows yeast-like buds and hyphae on 10% KOH preparation and has a pH of less than 4.5.

Treatment

Use miconazole or clotrimazole cream 200 mg intravaginally daily (qd) for 3 days in uncomplicated acute infections. Alternative therapy is one dose of fluconazole (Diflucan) 150 mg PO.

Prostatitis

■ NIH Classification System for Prostatitis Syndromes

Category I—Acute Bacterial Prostatitis

Acute bacterial prostatitis presents with sudden onset of chills, high fever, and low back and perineal pain. Patients have frequency, urgency, dysuria, and varying degrees of bladder outlet obstruction. Generalized malaise with arthralgias and myalgias is common. The prostate is exquisitely tender and swollen on digital rectal examination. Prostate massage should not be performed. The organism (usually *E. coli*) can generally be cultured from the voided urine.

TREATMENT A quinolone antibiotic such as ciprofloxacin (Cipro) 500 mg PO bid or levofloxacin (Levaquin) 500 mg PO qd is appropriate initial therapy. Patients should be treated for 4 to 6 weeks to prevent chronic infection. After 7 days of a quinolone, patients may be switched to TMP-SMX (Bactrim, Septra), 160 mg TMP and 800 mg SMX PO bid, for the remaining 3 to 5 weeks to keep cost down. Pathogen susceptibility should be checked from cultures. Bladder outlet obstruction must be managed appropriately.

Prostatic Abscess

Prostatic abscess is an uncommon complication of acute bacterial prostatitis. *E. coli* is thought to be responsible for 70% of cases; however, *N. gonorrhoeae* was the most common pathogen in the past. Patients present with acute retention, high fever, and a fluctuant prostate on rectal examination. Patients are frequently diabetic. CT scan of the pelvis or transrectal ultrasound can help make the diagnosis.

TREATMENT Treatment consists of antibiotics and surgical drainage by transperineal aspiration under local anesthesia with a large bore needle. A transurethral resection of the prostate (TURP) or perineal incision is occasionally necessary.

Category II—Chronic Bacterial Prostatitis

Chronic bacterial prostatitis has a variable presentation. It is caused by bacterial colonization of the prostatic ducts resulting in relapsing UTIs. Most patients present with lower urinary tract symptoms including frequency, urgency, and dysuria and some complaints of genital or perineal pain. Fever and chills are unusual. Recurring UTI caused by the same organism is the hallmark of chronic bacterial prostatitis. However, negative urine cultures do not exclude the diagnosis. Prostatic expressates show more than 10 WBCs per high power field (hpf) and macrophages containing fat (oval fat bodies). Prostatic calculi are often seen on plain films of the pelvis.

TREATMENT A quinolone antibiotic such as ciprofloxacin (Cipro) 500 mg PO bid or levofloxacin (Levaquin) 500 mg PO qd is effective therapy. Patients should be treated for 4 to 6 weeks. Alternatively, TMP-SMX (Bactrim, Septra), 160 mg TMP and 800 mg SMX PO bid, is also effective. Patients with prostatic calculi that are unresponsive to antibiotic therapy may benefit from a radical TURP.

Category III—Chronic Pelvic Pain Syndrome (CPPS)

The predominant symptom of CPPS is pain, usually in the perineum, suprapubic area, and penis. Pain with ejaculation is common, as is irritative and obstructive voiding symptoms including urgency, frequency, and hesitancy. Differentiation of subtypes IIIA from IIIB is the presence of inflammatory cells in the urine or expressed prostatic secretions (EPS).

Category IIIa—Chronic Nonbacterial Prostatitis

Chronic nonbacterial prostatitis is the most common prostatitis syndrome and has no known etiology. Possible causes include as yet unidentified pathogenic organisms or an intraprostatic urinary reflux causing a chemical prostatitis. Evidence suggests spastic dysfunction of the bladder neck and prostatic urethra from incomplete relaxation during voiding. This is thought to cause the intraprostatic urinary reflux. Patients present with irritative voiding symptoms and also complain of genital or perineal pain. Prostatic expressates will be positive for inflammatory cells (>15–20 WBCs per hpf), similar to chronic bacterial prostatitis. However, patients with nonbacterial prostatitis will have negative cultures and no history of documented UTIs.

TREATMENT α-Blockers have become the most important agents in the management of chronic nonbacterial prostatitis with the discovery of bladder neck–internal sphincter dyssynergia. Other symptomatic support includes antiinflammatory agents and hot sitz baths to help soothe painful symptomatic episodes. Patients are often given an initial round of antibiotics if there is confusion with chronic bacterial prostatitis.

Category IIIb—Prostatodynia

Prostatodynia describes a syndrome distinguished from nonbacterial prostatitis only by normal prostatic expressates. Prostatodynia describes patients who present with symptoms suggesting prostatitis but have negative cultures, no history of UTIs, and negative prostatic expressates for inflammation. These males are generally age 20 to 45 years and complain predominantly of perineal or pelvic pain, often associated with sitting or activity. The cause is unknown.

TREATMENT Management is identical to that for nonbacterial prostatitis.

Category IV—Asymptomatic Inflammatory Prostatitis

Category IV prostatitis does not cause symptoms; however, evidence of prostatic inflammation is demonstrated microscopically in EPS or histologic specimens.

Epididymitis and Orchitis

■ Acute Epididymitis

Acute epididymitis is an infection of the epididymis acquired by retrograde spread of organisms down the vas from the urethra or bladder. Patients present with heaviness and a dull, aching discomfort in the affected hemiscrotum that can radiate up to the ipsilateral flank. The epididymis will be markedly swollen and exquisitely tender to touch, eventually becoming a warm, red, enlarged, scrotal mass, indistinguishable from the testis. Fever and chills may develop, and patients usually have pyuria and bacteriuria.

Pathogens

In sexually active men younger than 35 years, *C. trachomatis* and *N. gonorrhoeae* are the most common organisms. In children and men older than 35 years, *E. coli* is the most common pathogen.

Diagnosis

Torsion of the testicle must always be ruled out. Torsion of the testicle is discussed in detail Chapter 10. The presence of epididymitis in children younger than 10 years is uncommon and should suggest urethral obstruction (e.g., stricture, valves, or meatal stenosis). Adult males are at risk of epididymitis from an indwelling Foley catheter and urethral instrumentation and after a TURP. Culture results are particularly important in this group. Sexually active males will usually have an accompanying urethritis. The diagnosis is usually made from history, physical examination, and positive urinalysis.

Treatment

Treatment should begin immediately. For sexually transmitted chlamydial or gonorrheal epididymitis, doxycycline 100 mg PO bid for 2 to 3 weeks or ofloxacin (Floxin) 300 mg PO bid is appropriate. For nonsexually transmitted episodes in older men and children TMP-SMX (Bactrim, Septra), 160 mg TMP and 800 mg SMX PO bid for 4 weeks, is recommended. Alternatively, a quinolone agent (ofloxacin or ciprofloxacin) is appropriate for both gram-negative and gonorrheal epididymitis. Antibiotic choices should be modified based on culture results. Management should include bedrest and scrotal elevation initially. Analgesics and a cord block with local anesthetic can provide considerable relief. Complete resolution of pain and swelling may take several weeks to months.

Abscess Formation

Abscess formation may complicate a prolonged episode of acute epididymitis. Fixation of the testis to the scrotal wall heralds such an event. An ultrasound should be obtained to confirm the presence of an abscess. Orchiectomy is usually indicated.

Chronic Epididymitis

Chronic epididymitis can be the result of several recurrent episodes of acute epididymitis producing chronic induration and pain. Treatment consists of long-term antibiotics or epididymectomy.

Orchitis

Orchitis is generally secondary to an extension of an associated epididymitis, producing an epididymo-orchitis. Treatment is identical to that for acute epididymitis.

■ **Mumps Orchitis**

Mumps orchitis is a specific instance of metastatic infection to the testis during an episode of viral mumps, usually occurring 4 to 6 days after the appearance of parotitis. Treatment consists of symptomatic relief, including bedrest, scrotal elevation, and analgesics. Mumps orchitis usually resolves spontaneously in 7 to 10 days.

GENITOURINARY TUBERCULOSIS

Pathogenesis

Genitourinary tuberculosis occurs secondary to prior pulmonary infection. Patients first inhale infected droplet nuclei that produce the primary lung infection, which manifests as a nonspecific bronchopneumonia and is often asymptomatic. Purified protein derivative (PPD) skin test will convert at this time, and the tubercle bacilli can become blood-borne, showering the kidney and occasionally the prostate. Renal infection progresses slowly, taking 15 to 20 years to destroy the kidney and producing little or no clinical disturbance until end stage. An abscess eventually invades a calyx, releasing WBCs and acid-fast bacteria (AFB) into the urine. Other genitourinary organ involvement occurs via this infected urine in most instances.

Presentation

Presentation is primarily that of irritative voiding symptoms with hematuria and sterile pyuria or tuberculous epididymitis unresponsive to antibiotics. Renal involvement is generally silent. The vas deferens may be thickened or beaded along with induration of the prostate or seminal vesicles. Vague generalized malaise, fatigue, and persistent low-grade fever or night sweats are characteristic. Patients will often give a prior history of pulmonary tuberculosis.

Diagnosis

Diagnosis is made by finding acid-fast bacteria in the urine or by urine cultures positive for *Mycobacterium tuberculosis*. Routine urine cultures are generally negative despite persistent pyuria. Workup should include CBC, chemistry panel, urinalysis, urine for acid-fast bacteria, urine for routine and tuberculosis culture, PPD skin test, chest radiograph, IVU, and cystoscopy. A negative tuberculin skin test makes diagnosis unlikely. An IV pyelogram may demonstrate the characteristic "moth eaten" appearance of the minor calyces.

Treatment

Use of a three-drug regimen is recommended for initial therapy: pyrazinamide 25 mg/kg body weight per day, isoniazid (INH) 300 mg PO qd, and rifampicin 450 mg PO qd for 4 months. Pyridoxine (vitamin B6) 25 mg/day should also be added to prevent the peripheral neuropathy occasionally seen with INH. Liver function tests should be monitored once a month when administering INH and rifampin. Streptomycin should be added if there is intense infection or severe bladder symptoms. Obstructive lesions in the kidney or ureters will require appropriate surgical therapy. Asymptomatic strictures in the lower third of the ureters may occur.

FUNGAL INFECTIONS (MYCOSES)

Fungal infections of the urinary tract are almost exclusively caused by C. *albicans* and occur usually in patients with one or more predisposing conditions, including central venous catheters, surgical drains, broad-spectrum antibiotics, steroids, cytotoxic agents, renal transplantation, indwelling Foley catheters, diabetes mellitus, malignancy, chronic debilitating diseases, and pregnancy. Renal metastases in a systemic fungal infection are common, occurring in up to 90% of patients with disseminated candidiasis.

Candidiasis

C. *albicans*, a yeastlike fungus, is a normal inhabitant of the intestinal tract (mainly the colon and oral cavity) and the vagina. It occurs in a unicellular form and as long threadlike pseudomycelia. The normal bacterial flora usually suppress its level of growth. Infection to the urinary tract can occur by either hematogenous (lymphatic or blood-borne) or retrograde (from anus to urethra) spread. The threadlike pseudomycelia of *Candida* tend to cluster, forming small bezoars or fungus balls that can cause ureteral obstruction.

■ Presentation

Presentation can range from asymptomatic candiduria or cystitis to pyelonephritis and septicemia. Pneumaturia can occur in diabetics because of fermentation of sugar in the urine.

■ Diagnosis

Diagnosis is based on positive cultures. Workup should include urinalysis, urine and blood cultures, IVU, and retrograde urograms if necessary. The urinary sediment will often make the diagnosis, showing yeast and mycelial forms. Urine specimens from females should be from a catheterized or aspirated sample. Bladder bezoars often produce a typical radiographic filling defect.

■ Treatment

Treatment should be based on the patient's total clinical picture and not just the presence of candiduria. Careful attention should be paid to controlling or eliminating any predisposing factors (i.e., remove or change central lines, drains, or Foley catheters; control diabetes; and eliminate broad-spectrum antibiotics). Fungus balls should be handled surgically as needed.

Asymptomatic Patients

The candiduria of asymptomatic patients will often resolve spontaneously. Treatment should be limited to controlling or eliminating any predisposing factors. Persistent candiduria warrants more aggressive treatment.

Candida Cystitis

Candida cystitis will usually respond to urinary alkalinization (pH 7.5) with sodium bicarbonate or bladder irrigation with amphotericin B (amphotericin B 50–100 mg in 1 L sterile water qd run over 12–24 hours via a three-way Foley catheter for 5–7 days). Alternatively, fluconazole (Diflucan) 200 mg PO qd for 10 days is effective.

Candida Vaginitis

Candida vaginitis can be treated with one 150-mg dose of fluconazole.

Seriously Ill Patients

Seriously ill patients should be started on immediate IV therapy with amphotericin B or fluconazole for 2 to 6 weeks. Monitor laboratory tests (CBC, chem-7, and liver function tests) every other day (qod). Amphotericin irrigation via cystostomy or nephrostomy tubes may be necessary.

Actinomycosis

Actinomycosis is a chronic granulomatous disease caused by the organism *Actinomyces israelii* (*A. bovis*). The disease will occasionally involve the kidneys, bladder, or testes. Marked fibrosis and spontaneous fistulae are characteristic. Diagnosis can be made by microscopic demonstration of the organism as yellow bodies called sulfur granules; however, culture results are usually necessary. Treatment consists of IV penicillin (20 million units/day for 2 weeks) or oral ampicillin (1,500 mg/day for 4 months). Surgical removal of the involved organ is occasionally necessary.

PARASITIC DISEASES

Schistosomiasis (Bilharziasis)

Schistosoma haematobium is a trematode or blood fluke endemic throughout most of Africa and the Middle East. It produces disease by following a life cycle that includes humans and an intermediate host. An increased incidence of squamous cell carcinoma of the bladder has been associated with schistosomal infection of the bladder. Presentation is classically that of hematuria and dysuria. Late clinical manifestations include bladder ulcers, stone formation, and silent obstructive uropathy.

Filariasis

The parasitic nematodes, *Wuchereria bancrofti* and *Brugia malayi*, are filarial worms about 0.5 cm long that live in human lymphatics. They are endemic in most tropical countries, and spread is by mosquitoes. Urogenital disease is the result of lymphatic filarial obstruction by adult worms. The tail of the epididymis and the lower spermatic cord are among the most common localization sites, causing funiculoepididymitis and elephantiasis of the penis, scrotum, or extremities.

Echinococcosis

The tapeworm *Echinococcus* is a primary parasite of the dog, with sheep and cattle as intermediary hosts. It is a disease primarily found in Australia, Argentina, and the Middle East where sheep-herding is common. *Echinococcus* eggs are passed via feces to their accidental host, humans, where they principally cause disease in the liver. However, 3% of cases involve the kidney. Hydatid cysts undergoing slow, concentric growth over many years are the pathologic lesions. They present as a renal mass, often calcified on plain films, and may be asymptomatic or cause symptoms of dull flank pain. CT and IVU can make the diagnosis. Treatment is surgical excision; usually a nephrectomy is elected. Needle aspiration is unwise.

ANTIBIOTICS COMMONLY USED IN UROLOGY

The essence of treating an infectious disease is the isolation and identification of the pathogenic organism and determination of its sensitivity to antimicrobial agents. However, because of the necessary delay in obtaining these results, patients must be treated based on other less exacting clinical evidence. Therefore, it is fundamental to have a specific working knowledge of the various antibiotic choices available and an understanding of their mode of action and possible adverse side effects.

General Guidelines for Antibiotic Therapy

1. Obtain all culture specimens before initiating therapy.
2. Be alert to host deficiencies such as malnutrition, chronic alcoholism, renal failure, impaired circulation, and immunosuppression.
3. Consider hospital-acquired bacterial resistances.
4. Remove foreign materials, debride necrotic tissue, drain abscesses, and relieve obstruction.
5. Use IV administration for serious infections, at least initially.
6. Adjust antibiotic dosages as necessary for renal or hepatic dysfunction.
7. Monitor therapy (i.e., temperature curve, WBC count, signs of inflammation, and follow-up cultures).
8. Select agents based on their potential toxicity and the severity of the infection.
9. Control antibiotic resistance:
   a. Only use antibiotics when necessary.
   b. Avoid use of newer agents when available agents are effective.
   c. Wash hands after seeing each patient.
10. Revise antibiotic choice to reflect culture and sensitivity results.

Sulfonamides

Sulfonamides (SMX) act by inhibiting the uptake of paraamino-benzoic acid and thus inhibit the synthesis of tetrahydrofolic acid, necessary for subsequent DNA synthesis. Mammalian cells do not produce folic acid and, consequently, are unaffected. Sulfonamides are bacteriostatic on most routine coliform bacteria. Negative side effects include allergic reactions, rash, fever, renal and liver damage, blood dyscrasia, and vasculitis. Dosage is sulfisoxazole 2 to 4 g/day PO.

Trimethoprim

Trimethoprim (TMP) also inhibits synthesis of tetrahydrofolic acid by competitive inhibition of the enzyme dihydrofolate reductase. It is bacteriostatic for many common urinary pathogens such as *E. coli*, *Proteus*, *Klebsiella*, and *Enterobacter*. It is a good choice for urinary prophylaxis because of a low incidence of resistance (10%) when used this way. Negative side effects include rash, fever, and hematologic and gastrointestinal abnormalities. Dosage is 100 mg every 12 hours (q12h) PO.

Trimethoprim-Sulfamethoxazole (Bactrim, Septra)

TMP-SMX is a fixed dose combination of 80 mg TMP and 400 mg SMX that together is bactericidal for most common urinary pathogens. It is also available in a double-strength tablet of 160 mg TMP and 800 mg SMX. Negative side effects include rash, fever, gastrointestinal symptoms (nausea, vomiting, diarrhea), and blood dyscrasia. Dosage is two regular tablets q12h PO.

Penicillins

Penicillins inhibit bacterial cell wall synthesis (bactericidal) by irreversible binding of the β-lactam ring to the enzyme transpeptidase. Bacterial resistance is observed in those bacteria (most often *S. aureus*) that produce β-lactamase, an enzyme that breaks the β-lactam ring. Penicillins are excreted intact by the kidneys (primarily tubular secretion). Probenecid blocks tubular secretion and therefore enhances serum levels. Negative side effects include allergic reactions, rash, diarrhea, and anaphylaxis.

- *Natural penicillin*—penicillin G (benzyl penicillin) and penicillin V potassium

- *Synthetic penicillins*—ampicillin, amoxicillin, carbenicillin (Geocillin), and ticarcillin (Ticar)
- *Synthetic β-lactamase-resistant penicillins*—methicillin, oxacillin, cloxacillin, dicloxacillin, and nafcillin

Cephalosporins

Cephalosporins are also β-lactam antibiotics like penicillin with a wide antibacterial spectrum and resistance to some β-lactamase-producing bacteria. They are excreted in the urine mainly by tubular secretion. First-generation cephalosporins have good gram-positive activity, except with group D streptococci (enterococcus) and methicillin-resistant *S. aureus*, whereas second- and third-generation agents have increasing activity against gram-negatives with less gram-positive effectiveness. Negative side effects include allergic reactions, rash, fever, anaphylaxis, and synergistic toxicity with aminoglycosides. Cross-reactivity with penicillin-allergic patients occasionally occurs.

- *First generation*—cephalothin (Keflin), cefazolin (Ancef, Kefzol), cephapirin (Cefadyl), cephradine (Velosef, Anspor), cephalexin (Keflex), and cefadroxil (Duricef)
- *Second generation*— cefuroxime (Zinacef), cefaclor (Ceclor), and cefoxitin (Mefoxin)
- *Third generation*—cefotaxime (Claforan), ceftizoxime (Cefizox), ceftriaxone (Rocephin), ceftazidime (Fortaz, Tazicef), and cefoperazone (Cefobid)
- *Oral cephalosporins*—cephalexin (Keflex), cephradine (Velosef), cefadroxil (Duricef), and cefaclor (Ceclor)

Aminoglycosides

Aminoglycosides are a group of bactericidal antibiotics that act by inhibiting bacterial protein synthesis. They are active against most gram-negative urinary tract pathogens including *E. coli*, *Enterobacter*, *Klebsiella*, *Proteus*, *Pseudomonas*, and *Serratia*. The drug is excreted in the urine by glomerular filtration. Negative side effects include ototoxicity and nephrotoxicity (nonoliguric renal failure after 5–10 days of therapy). Nephrotoxicity is potentiated by hypovolemia, cephalosporins, and furosemide (Lasix). Serum levels should be monitored and adjusted for renal insufficiency. Peak levels (taken 30–60 minutes after infusion) should be in the range of 4 to 6 μg/mL. Trough levels (taken just before the next dose) should be greater than 2 μg/mL.

Gentamicin or tobramycin is a good first choice for most serious gram-negative infections. Amikacin is effective for gentamicin- or tobramycin-resistant organisms.

Tetracyclines

Tetracyclines are bacteriostatic antibiotics that interfere with bacterial protein synthesis. Excretion in the urine is mainly by glomerular filtration. Negative side effects include allergic reactions, phototoxicity, nausea, vomiting, diarrhea, superinfections, hepatic toxicity, and staining of the teeth in children. Gastrointestinal absorption is decreased if taken with food [tetracycline, doxycycline (Vibramycin), and minocycline (Minocin)].

Erythromycin

Erythromycin is a macrolide antibiotic that inhibits bacterial protein synthesis. It is effective against *Mycoplasma*, *Ureaplasma*, and *Chlamydia*. Negative side effects include allergic reactions, cholestatic hepatitis, and epigastric distress. Dosage is 0.5 to 1.0 g q6h PO/IV.

Clindamycin (Cleocin)

Clindamycin inhibits bacterial protein synthesis and is effective against most gram-positive organisms and anaerobic infections, including *Bacteroides fragilis*. Negative side effects include gastrointestinal disturbances, mostly diarrhea and pseudomembranous enterocolitis secondary to *Clostridium difficile*. Dosage is 300 to 900 mg IV q6h (adjust dosage for hepatic dysfunction).

Vancomycin (Vancocin)

Vancomycin is a bactericidal antibiotic that inhibits cell wall synthesis. It is active against gram-positive bacteria and C. *difficile* and is excreted by the kidneys unchanged. Negative side effects include ototoxicity, fever, phlebitis, and nephrotoxicity. Dosage is 500 mg IV q12h (adjust dosage for renal insufficiency).

Metronidazole (Flagyl)

Metronidazole is a bactericidal antibiotic for anaerobic infections of gram-negative organisms, especially *B. fragilis*. It acts by inhibiting DNA synthesis. Other therapeutic uses include amebiasis, giardiasis, and vaginitis secondary to *Trichomonas* or *Gardnerella*. It is eliminated primarily by hepatic metabolism. Negative side effects include nausea, vomiting, diarrhea, neurologic symptoms, and a sulfiram (Antabuse)-like effect when taken with alcohol. Dosage is 500 mg PO tid.

Quinolones

The quinolones are a class of bactericidal antibiotics that inhibit bacterial DNA synthesis (DNA gyrase). They have a broad spectrum of coverage including most gram-negative and gram-positive organisms, particularly *Pseudomonas* and group D streptococcus. They should be reserved for patients with complicated UTIs unresponsive to other oral agents. *Quinolones should not be used in children or pregnant females*. Use of quinolones should generally be avoided or monitored in patients on warfarin (Coumadin).

■ Ciprofloxacin (Cipro)

Ciprofloxacin has increased activity against *P. aeruginosa*, *Providencia rettgeri*, *Acinetobacter spp.*, and *S. aureus* and has better pharmacokinetic properties than norfloxacin. It can be given intravenously, as well as orally, on a twice-daily regimen. Negative side effects include skin rash, gastrointestinal complaints, headache, vertigo, and malaise. Potential drug interactions have been reported when used with other drugs that utilize the cytochrome P-450 enzyme system. Ciprofloxacin should be avoided in patients taking theophylline because of fatal reactions reported and patients on warfarin (Coumadin) because of increased INR. Dosage is 250 to 500 mg PO/IV bid.

■ Levofloxacin (Levaquin)

Levofloxacin is an L-isomer of ofloxacin with similar broad-spectrum coverage and bioavailability but with decreased side effects of ofloxacin. Dosage is 500 mg PO/IV qd.

Other Quinolones

Other quinolones include moxifloxacin (Avelox) and lomefloxacin (Maxaquin).

URINARY ANTISEPTICS

Nitrofurantoin (Macrobid)

Nitrofurantoin is a synthetic bacteriocidal agent *only* effective in the urine where therapeutic levels are achieved. Never use in treating tissue infections such as pyelonephritis or prostatitis. Many urinary pathogens are sensitive; however, *Proteus* and *Pseudomonas* are usually resistant. Nitrofurantoin is useful for the prophylaxis of recurrent lower UTIs. Resistant bacterial strains rarely emerge during long-term use. Negative side effects include gastrointestinal upset, hypersensitivity reactions, rashes, pulmonary infiltrates, and hemolytic anemia in glucose-6-phosphate dehydrogenase–deficient patients. Dosage is 100 mg q12h PO.

Methenamine (Mandelate—Mandelamine, Hippurate—Hiprex)

Methenamine is a condensation product of formaldehyde and ammonia that releases the formaldehyde in acid urine. Its bacteriostatic property is only effective in acid urine (pH less than 6.0). Ascorbic acid (vitamin C) is often given to help acidify the urine. Methenamine is combined with mandelic acid or hippuric acid to promote an acid urine and to enhance its antibacterial effect. Chronic long-term suppression of UTIs is its only use. Negative side effects include gastrointestinal distress and crystalluria. Dosage is 1 g q6h (Mandelamine) and 1 g q12h (Hiprex) PO [ascorbic acid 0.5 to 2 g every 4 hours (q4h); titrate to urinary pH].

ANTIBIOTIC PROPHYLAXIS

Wound Classification

1. *Clean*—respiratory, gastrointestinal, or genitourinary tracts not entered
2. *Clean contaminated*—respiratory, gastrointestinal, or genitourinary tracts entered without excessive contaminated spillage
3. *Contaminated*—area of nonpurulent inflammation entered or a major break in sterile technique
4. *Dirty*—trauma more than 4 hours old, gross pus, or a perforated viscus

General Recommendations

1. Culture urine before surgery.
2. Sterilize urine before any elective surgery.
3. Select an antibiotic that gives high urine and urinary tract tissue concentrations.
4. Short-term prophylactic antibiotic regimens are preferred to minimize development of resistance (e.g., 24–48 hours).
5. Patients with preoperative indwelling Foley catheters or mature nephrostomy tracts should receive prophylactic antibiotics.
6. For an antibacterial agent to be effective, it must be present in the tissues at the time the incision is made, so start prophylaxis before incision (i.e., on-call).
7. Patients with increased risk of infective complications (e.g., diabetics, renal failure, neurogenic bladder, and immunosuppressed patients) should receive prophylactic antibiotics.

Prophylaxis Recommended (Sterile Urine)

1. Surgery involving the use of bowel—an oral bowel preparation (i.e., erythromycin base and neomycin) and systemic antibiotics
2. Penile prostheses or artificial urinary sphincters
3. Transrectal needle biopsy (cleansing enema and systemic antibiotic)
4. Patients at high risk for developing bacterial endocarditis (suspected congenital or acquired heart disease, prosthetic valves, prior history of infective endocarditis, ventriculoseptal patches, mitral valve prolapse, and transvenous pacemakers)
5. Surgery of infected calculi
6. TURP or transurethral resection of bladder tumors

Prophylaxis Against Reinfection

Oral antibiotic therapy can produce resistant strains in the fecal flora with subsequent resistant UTIs. The following agents have been demonstrated to be useful when long-term prophylactic therapy is indicated: TMP-SMX, nitrofurantoin, and TMP alone.

SEPTIC SHOCK

Septic shock is a condition characterized by abnormal circulatory function secondary to overwhelming infection. The urinary tract is a common site of origin. Gram-negative sepsis is most common with *E. coli*, accounting for about 20% of all cases. Mortality rate has been reported to be as high as 50%.

Pathophysiology and Clinical Manifestations

The prime initiator of gram-negative septic shock is endotoxin, a lipopolysaccharide component of the bacterial cell wall. Lipopolysaccharide-stimulated monocytes release cytokines such as tumor necrosis factor and interleukin-1. Profound tissue hypoxia is a cardinal feature. Two distinct phases of septic shock are usually noted: (a) the initial hyperdynamic state or warm shock is characterized by increased cardiac output, decreased peripheral vascular resistance, low central venous pressure, and warm extremities; eventually cardiac decompensation will result in (b) the hypodynamic state or cold shock, which is characterized by decreased cardiac output, increased peripheral vascular resistance, and cool extremities. Fever, leukocytosis, and a profound metabolic acidosis are usual.

Diagnosis

Septic shock presents initially as altered mental status, hyperventilation, and respiratory alkalosis. It can easily be confused with other conditions, and a high index of suspicion must be maintained. Differential diagnosis includes atelectasis, pulmonary embolus, pneumonia, acute hemorrhage, and myocardial infarction. Workup should begin with history, physical examination, urinalysis, CBC, and electrolytes. Patients should be pan-cultured, including blood, urine, sputum, and wounds, before starting antibiotic therapy. Arterial blood gases and serum lactate dehydrogenase levels should be carefully followed. Chest radiograph is mandatory, and plain films of the abdomen and CT scan, IVU, or renal ultrasound may help identify the source of infection.

Management Guidelines

The most important aspect of management is to eliminate the source of infection.
1.   Drain abscess; relieve obstructive uropathy; and, if necessary, debride wounds.

2. Start appropriate antibiotic therapy immediately, without waiting for culture results.
3. Place a central line for access and monitoring the central venous pressure.
4. Do not hesitate to float a Swan-Ganz catheter if the hemodynamic condition is in question.
5. Use normal saline for fluid resuscitation.
6. Avoid overcorrection of metabolic acidosis because this will rapidly resolve after restoring adequate perfusion.
7. Use dopamine if pressor agents are needed to support the circulation. Mix 400 mg dopamine in 250 mL D5W, start infusion at 2 μg/kg per minute (5 mL/hour for a 70-kg adult), and titrate to blood pressure.
8. Digitalization may be useful for patients in obvious cardiac failure.
9. Large doses of corticosteroids may be helpful.
10. Intubation with mechanical ventilation and positive end-expiratory pressure are important for patients developing respiratory failure and shock lung.
11. Monitor patient's progression with arterial blood gases and serum lactate.

18 Sexually Transmitted Diseases

The incidence, prevalence, and variety of sexually transmitted diseases have increased remarkably in recent years. These include the five classic venereal diseases (gonorrhea, syphilis, chancroid, lymphogranuloma venereum, and granuloma inguinale), together with urethritis, vaginitis, hepatitis, genital herpes virus, and acquired immunodeficiency syndrome (AIDS). Serious consequences of these diseases have also increased: spontaneous abortions, ectopic pregnancies, pelvic inflammatory disease, infertility, cervical carcinoma, and death. Additionally, 60% of patients who have one sexually transmitted disease have been shown to have another. In light of these facts, examination and treatment of all sexual partners are strongly recommended.

NONGONOCOCCAL URETHRITIS

Chlamydia trachomatis is believed to be the most common cause of nonspecific urethritis in males (followed by *Ureaplasma urealyticum*, *Mycoplasma hominis*, and *Trichomonas vaginalis*). It has a prolonged incubation of 5 to 21 days and produces a watery or mucoid, whitish discharge with or without dysuria.

Diagnosis

Diagnosis of nongonococcal urethritis requires exclusion of gonorrhea and demonstration of urethritis (Gram stain of urethral swab showing more than four polymorphonucleocytes per oil immersion field). Confirmation with chlamydial culture should be attempted.

Treatment

Azithromycin 1 g orally (PO) in a single dose, doxycycline 100 mg PO twice a day (bid) for 7 days, or ofloxacin (Floxin) 300 mg PO bid for 7 days is appropriate for chlamydia or *U. urealyticum*. If *T. vaginalis* is suspected, then metronidazole 2 g PO in a single dose or 250 mg PO three times a day (tid) for 7 days should be given.

Reiter's Syndrome

Reiter's syndrome is a rare complication of nongonococcal urethritis caused by *C. trachomatis*, which presents with arthritis, conjunctivitis, balanitis circinata, or keratodermia blennorrhagia.

GONORRHEA

Gonorrhea is caused by a gram-negative intracellular diplococcus, *Neisseria gonorrhoeae*. It has a short incubation of 2 to 8 days and most often produces a purulent, yellowish, urethral discharge with dysuria. (Up to 45% of males with gonococcal urethritis will also be infected with *C. trachomatis*.) Complications of gonorrhea in males include epididymitis, prostatitis, seminal vesiculitis, and urethral strictures.

Diagnosis

Diagnosis is based on a history of sexual contact, a purulent discharge with dysuria, and a positive Gram stain (intracellular gram-negative diplococci within polymorphonuclear leukocytes) and/or culture. The specimen for culture and the Gram stain must be carefully taken from within the urethra using a calcium alginate urethrogenital swab (Calgiswab) at least 1 hour after the patient last voided. A modified Thayer-Martin culture medium should be directly inoculated followed by prompt incubation. After culture inoculation, the swab should be rolled onto a clean microscope slide that is then air dried, heat fixed, and Gram stained. The presence of intracellular gram-negative diplococci makes the diagnosis. Routine urine cultures should also be obtained.

Treatment

Treatment should not await culture results even if the Gram stain is negative when suspicion is high. Appropriate regimens include ceftriaxone 250 mg intramuscularly (IM), ciprofloxacin 500 mg PO, or ofloxacin 400 mg PO. *Chlamydia* coverage is also recommended with doxycycline 100 mg PO bid for 7 days.

SYPHILIS

The spirochete *Treponema pallidum* is the causative pathogen in syphilis. It usually gains entrance through the intact skin or mucous membranes of the penis. Syphilis has been called the "great imitator" because of its varied manifestations as it progresses through defined stages.

Primary syphilis is characterized by the chancre, a painless, shallow ulcer with indurated borders that appears 10 to 30 days following infection. It generally is solitary and lasts for 1 to 5 weeks.

Secondary syphilis is characterized by highly infectious macular papular or papulosquamous skin eruptions involving the palms and soles, the oral cavity, and the anogenital areas with generalized adenopathy.

Latent syphilis is without signs or symptoms of the disease; however, the spirochete has persisted in the body and has invaded all organs, most characteristically the cardiovascular and central nervous systems (e.g., tabes dorsalis). The patient remains potentially infectious for approximately the first 2 years of the disease.

Diagnosis

Identification of the spirochete by darkfield microscopic examination of fresh material from a chancre is diagnostic. Positive rapid plasma reagin test, which is replacing the VDRL (Venereal Disease Research Laboratory), is serologic evidence of syphilis. Serologic titers develop between 3 weeks and 3 months after infection. It is almost 100% positive in secondary syphilis. The fluorescent treponema antibody-absorption (FTA-ABS) test is the most specific and sensitive test available for syphilis.

Treatment

Benzathine penicillin G 2.4×10^6 units IM in a single dose is the drug of choice for primary, secondary, or latent syphilis of less than 1 year. Doxycycline 100 mg PO bid or tetracycline 500 mg PO four times a day (qid) for 15 days is an alternative for penicillin-allergic patients.

CHANCROID

Chancroid or soft chancre is caused by *Haemophilus ducreyi*, a gram-negative rod that enters abraded skin or mucous membranes, usually during coitus. It has a short incubation of 1 to 5 days and can spread by autoinoculation. Its clinical features are soft, painful, dirty, malodorous penile ulcers, often associated with tender, unilateral, matted inguinal adenopathy. Chancroid must be differentiated from syphilis, lymphogranuloma venereum, and granuloma inguinale.

Diagnosis

Diagnosis is often made clinically; however, attempts to culture the organism should be made despite the difficulty of doing so. A Gram stain smear from the base of the ulcer may show gram-negative coccobacilli in chains with a "school of fish" appearance.

Treatment

Ceftriaxone 250 mg IM once or erythromycin 500 mg PO qid for 7 days is effective. An alternative regimen is ciprofloxacin 500 PO bid for 3 days or trimethoprim-sulfamethoxazole DS (160/800) PO bid for 7 days. Fluctuant inguinal abscesses should be drained by aspiration rather than incision to avoid a chronic discharging sinus.

LYMPHOGRANULOMA VENEREUM

Lymphogranuloma venereum is caused by the obligate intracellular organism C. trachomatis and is acquired primarily during coitus. It has an incubation of 1 to 12 weeks, resulting in a painless primary papule, erosion, or vesicular lesion that heals quickly. Eventually, unilateral inguinal adenopathy appears with matted nodes fixed to the skin that will ultimately drain purulent exudate through multiple sinus tracts. Extension to deep perirectal pelvic nodes can result in proctitis and rectal strictures. Fistulae involving the rectum, bladder, and vagina can arise.

Diagnosis

Diagnosis is usually made on clinical grounds by exclusion of syphilis, chancroid, and granuloma inguinale or by culture of C. trachomatis. The Frei test is no longer used.

Treatment

Doxycycline 100 mg PO bid for 21 days or tetracycline or erythromycin 500 mg PO qid for 3 weeks is recommended. Fluctuant lymph nodes should be drained by aspiration and not incision to avoid chronic draining fistulae.

GRANULOMA INGUINALE

Granuloma inguinale is caused by the gram-negative rod *Calymmatobacterium granulomatis*, also referred to as Donovan's body. Its exact mode of transmission is unknown; however, it generally presents as a hypertrophic genital lesion with rolled, everted, and raised edges and has been associated with sexual contact. The pathologic lesion is the result of hypertrophic granulation tissue that bleeds easily and often involves the inguinal nodes. An association with squamous cell carcinoma has been noted.

Diagnosis

Diagnosis requires demonstration of Donovan's body, usually within large mononuclear cells, by Wright- or Giemsa-stained smears of scrapings or biopsy specimens. A biopsy must be performed to rule out carcinoma.

Treatment

Tetracycline or erythromycin 500 mg PO qid for 3 weeks or trimethoprim-sulfamethoxazole (one double strength PO bid) is the treatment of choice.

CONDYLOMATA ACUMINATA (VENEREAL WARTS)

Condyloma acuminatum is a wartlike papilloma or cauliflower-like lesion of the skin caused by a human papillomavirus (HPV) and is transmitted by direct sexual contact. HPV is strongly associated with cervical cancer and cancer of the penis. The goal of treatment is removal of exophytic warts and resolution of signs and symptoms but not eradication of HPV. No therapy has been shown to eradicate HPV; thus, there is no benefit in treating patients with subclinical HPV infection.

Presentation

Condylomata are typically found on the external genitalia but may also occur in the urethra. Patients with urethral involvement will often have visible lesions around the meatus. Hematuria and irritative symptoms, including frequency and dysuria, are common signs and symptoms suggesting intraurethral lesions in males with visible warts.

Diagnosis

Identification of visible lesions is straightforward. Biopsy and examination of the histopathology of larger lesions should be considered. Cystourethroscopy should be performed if intraurethral involvement is suspected. Use of 5% acetic acid painted on the external genitalia may show subclinical, flat condylomata appearing as whitish areas; however, the usefulness of this is unclear.

Treatment

Mucocutaneous condylomata acuminata are most common and are best treated by cryotherapy with liquid nitrogen or direct application of 10% to 25% podophyllin in tincture of benzoin or 50% trichloracetic acid (TCA). The podophyllin must be washed off within 6 hours to prevent serious irritation. TCA can be painful, and use of 5% lidocaine/prilocaine (EMLA) cream before application of TCA can be helpful. Excision with scissors and local anesthesia cream (EMLA) is a simple surgical option for small lesions. More extensive lesions can be managed by laser ablation. Less than 5% of patients will develop urethral disease, 90% of which will involve only the external meatus and distal penile urethra. If only a few lesions are noted within the urethra and none is circumferential, then excision or fulguration with a resectoscope or Bugbee electrode is appropriate. When extensive or circumferential areas of the urethra are involved, daily instillation of 5-fluorouracil cream (5% Efudex) with a cone-tip applicator for 7 days is recommended. Particularly severe or persistent cases may necessitate exteriorization of the urethra, for application of podophyllin, with a second-stage urethroplasty. (Podophyllin should not be used intraurethrally.)

The most frequent complication of all condylomata acuminata is recurrence or reinfection; 10% to 25% podophyllin in benzoin,

TCA 50%, or bichloracetic acid should all be applied in the physician's office. Some questions have been raised about prolonged use of crude podophyllin and carcinogenesis.

Home Therapy

Podofilox gel (Condylox) is 0.5% podophyllin—apply bid for 3 days/week for up to 4 weeks (do not use if patient is pregnant). Apply imiquimod cream (Aldara) at bedtime (qhs) for 3 days per week for up to 16 weeks.

GENITAL HERPES SIMPLEX

Herpes simplex virus (HSV) infection occurs by direct inoculation of skin or mucosal surfaces. Two species of HSV exist: HSV type I (oral) and HSV type II (genital). Both can infect genital or oral regions. HSV travels up sensory nerve roots and establishes a latent infection in the dorsal root ganglion. Viral shedding occurs primarily from ruptured vesicular skin lesions but also can occur during asymptomatic periods.

Presentation

Primary infections will often have systemic symptoms including fever, headaches, malaise, myalgias, or lymphadenopathy. Urinary retention secondary to local pain or sacral radiculopathy is not uncommon. Recurrent infections are generally less severe and are manifested primarily by the characteristic skin lesions (grouped vesicles, erosions, and/or crusted lesions) lasting 4 to 15 days.

Diagnosis

Cytologic diagnosis by Papanicolaou smear demonstrating intranuclear inclusions or viral culture is most effective. The Tzanck cytologic smear of skin lesions is quick and effective when positive; however, a negative result should be followed up by direct immunofluorescence with anti-HSV antibodies. Serologic tests cannot prove active disease, only previous viral exposure. A negative serologic test rules out infection.

Treatment

Oral famciclovir has replaced acyclovir. It is not virucidal or curative, but it does block viral replication and is clinically effective in
treating primary and recurrent infections by decreasing their
severity, frequency, and duration. Famciclovir 125 mg PO for 5
days is given tid for first episodes and bid for recurrences.

ACQUIRED IMMUNODEFICIENCY SYNDROME

The urologist is unlikely to play a major role in managing AIDS;
however, urologic consultations will occur. It is wise for all
physicians to keep abreast of current information about this
rapidly evolving disease.

Etiology

The etiologic agent in AIDS is the human immunodeficiency virus
(HIV). The HIV retrovirus affects primarily the helper T
lymphocytes (CD4+ T cells), causing depletion of CD4+ T cells
and impaired immunologic function. HIV infection can produce a
spectrum of clinical manifestations ranging from asymptomatic
infection to severe immunodeficiency and neurologic disease. The
virus is spread by sexual contact with an infected individual,
sharing a contaminated needle, and receipt of infected blood or
blood products and transmission from mother to unborn child.

Blood Transfusions

All blood is tested for the presence of anti-HIV antibodies by
enzyme-linked immunosorbent assay (ELISA), and all units
testing positive are discarded. ELISA was purposefully designed to
be sensitive to minimize false negatives; however, this has resulted
in a high false positive rate of up to 90%. ELISA positive units are
tested by Western blot electrophoresis for confirmation of anti-
HIV antibodies and detection of viral core or envelope antigens
before notifying the donor. Unfortunately, transfusion-associated
HIV infection from a seronegative donor can occur and has been
reported. Patients undergoing surgery should be informed of the
risk of AIDS. The use of autologous blood transfusion should be
made available for elective surgery.

19 Benign Prostatic Hyperplasia

Benign prostatic hyperplasia (BPH) is characterized by progressive enlargement of the prostate gland resulting in bladder outlet obstruction and increasingly difficult voiding. It is a disease of the elderly, rarely affecting males younger than age 40. The mean age at which patients develop symptoms is between 60 and 65 years.

PATHOGENESIS

The prostate consists of three distinct zones: an outer peripheral zone, a central zone, and a periurethral transition zone. BPH develops in the transition zone, whereas prostate cancer usually arises in the peripheral zone. Clinically, the prostate is still often considered to have five lobes: anterior, posterior, median, and two lateral lobes.

The cause of BPH remains unclear; however, its relationship to aging and the testes is well documented. Most current theories on the etiology of BPH focus on an increased sensitivity to androgens and a decreased rate of cell death. Direct stromal-epithelial interaction under hormonal control appears to be essential to the process.

Prostate growth and development are under the influence of the male hormone, testosterone, and its more active metabolite dihydrotestosterone (DHT). Testosterone, which is produced primarily by the testes under control of the hypothalamic-pituitary axis, is converted to DHT by the enzyme 5-α-reductase. DHT is the major intracellular androgen and is believed to be responsible for the maintenance of BPH. With advancing age, Leydig cell testosterone production decreases, resulting in a relative excess of estrogens. Estrogens have been demonstrated to cause increased nuclear accumulation of DHT receptors and to result in a net increased formation of DHT within the prostate. DHT stimulation results in increased production of epidermal growth factor (EGF), whereas other factors cause a reduction in programmed cell death or apoptosis, presumably as a result of transforming growth factor-β (TGF-β). BPH is believed to result from the imbalance of stromal and epithelial hyperplasia caused by EGF in the face of reduced apoptosis caused by TGF-β.

PATHOPHYSIOLOGY

Prostatic hyperplasia would be of no importance were it not for the consequent bladder outlet obstruction. The pathophysiology of bladder outlet obstruction has three components: a mechanical component, a dynamic component, and the detrusor response.

Mechanical Obstruction

With progressive prostatic growth, patients will present clinically with lateral and/or median lobe enlargement. As prostatic enlargement encroaches on the urethra, urinary outflow obstruction occurs. The mechanical component of obstruction is a direct result of this enlarging mass of tissue and its ability to increase outlet resistance and obstruct urine flow. The outer prostate glands proper become compressed against the prostatic capsule during this growth, resulting in a thick pseudocapsule referred to as the surgical capsule.

The anatomic configuration of the prostate can have an important effect on the degree of obstruction produced. Some patients can develop primarily median lobe hyperplasia or just a hyperplastic posterior commissure of the bladder neck, which is commonly referred to as a median bar. In these settings, relatively small degrees of hyperplasia can result in major impairment of flow. The enlarging mass of hyperplastic tissue and the favorable or unfavorable anatomic configuration it takes are usually the major components of prostatic obstruction. The overall size of the prostate in BPH often correlates poorly with the degree of obstructive symptoms but can be predictive of the success or failure of various treatment modalities.

Dynamic Obstruction—Prostate Smooth Muscle

The dynamic component of prostatic obstruction is related to the tone of the prostatic smooth muscle fibers. Smooth muscle fibers constitute a significant component of the true capsule, intervening stroma within the prostate, periurethral area, and the bladder neck.

Smooth muscle fibers of the prostate and bladder neck are richly innervated by adrenergic fibers of the sympathetic nervous system and α_1-type receptors. Specifically α_{1A}-subtype receptors predominate within the prostate, whereas α_{1B}-receptors mediate peripheral vasoconstriction. The baseline tone of the sympathetic autonomic nervous system is believed to modulate these smooth muscle fibers and, thus, prostatic urethral resistance. Medications containing adrenergic agonists (e.g., nasal decongestants) can result in worsening outlet obstruction or urinary retention. α-Adrenergic blockers are effectively used to relax prostatic smooth muscle and thus lower bladder outlet resistance.

Detrusor Response

As outlet resistance increases, the bladder responds by increasing its force of contraction. By developing increased intravesical voiding pressures, the bladder can maintain flow and the appearance of normalcy. The added work to overcome outlet resistance results in detrusor hypertrophy, hyperplasia, and deposition of collagen within the bladder wall. This results in what is seen at cystoscopy as trabeculation, cellules, and diverticula. With thickening of the bladder wall, its normal elasticity is lost and compliance decreases. The loss of compliance results in a decrease in the functional capacity of the bladder, i.e., increased intravesical pressure for a given volume. These bladder changes also cause the development of detrusor instability, or loss of normal control over the reflex detrusor response.

Early in the course of obstruction, the bladder is able to compensate. However, with progression, irritative voiding symptoms (e.g., frequency, urgency, nocturia, and urgency incontinence) result. It is the irritative voiding symptoms that are most responsible for the patient's complaints. Untreated, this process can progress to severe bladder decompensation and dilatation, ureterovesical obstruction and hydroureteronephrosis, and, ultimately, renal insufficiency.

DIAGNOSIS

Presentation/History

BPH is characterized by a spectrum of lower urinary tract symptoms (LUTS) previously referred to as prostatism:
- Decreased force and caliber of stream
- Hesitancy and straining to void
- Interruption of stream
- Postvoid dribbling
- Sensation of incomplete emptying
- Frequency and nocturia
- Urinary retention (acute or chronic)

LUTS (see Chapter 2) encompass both obstructive and irritative symptoms. Obstructive (voiding) symptoms (e.g., slow, weak stream) are a direct result of the increased outflow resistance, whereas irritative (storage) symptoms (e.g., frequency, urgency, nocturia) are secondary to bladder instability because of detrusor hypertrophy. Obstructive symptoms are the key feature. Irritative symptoms without obstructive symptoms are unlikely to be due to BPH. If irritative symptoms are the principal complaint, be alert for bladder cancer, infection, stones, or neurogenic bladder (such as Parkinson's disease or stroke) as the etiology. Exclude other causes of similar LUTS, such as polyuria from diabetes or congestive heart failure, history of urethral strictures, or medications (anticholinergics, antidepressants, or nasal decongestants).

A detailed and careful history and symptom assessment are critical. Symptom assessment can be enhanced by use of the International Prostate Symptom Score (IPSS) and the BPH Impact Index (BII). The IPSS is a data collection tool consisting of seven questions for the patient that quantitate his symptom severity. The maximum score is 35. A score of 0 to 8 is regarded as mild, 9 to 19 as moderate, and 20 or above as severe. BII quantifies how bothersome the symptoms are.

Differential Diagnosis

- Bladder cancer
- Infection (cystitis or prostatitis)
- Bladder stones
- Neurogenic (Parkinson's disease, stroke, dementia, multiple sclerosis, spinal cord injury, etc.)
- Prostate cancer
- Bladder neck contracture or urethral stricture
- Medications (anticholinergics, antidepressants, decongestants, etc.)

Workup

■ Physical Examination

The digital rectal examination (DRE) is important. Carefully palpate the prostate, paying attention to size, shape, and consistency. Any suspicious areas (see Chapter 3) should be biopsied. The patient's symptoms are a better indication of the degree of obstruction than the size of the gland on DRE; however, a large prostate increases the risk for acute urinary retention. Examine the lower abdomen for evidence of a palpable bladder. Examine the penis for evidence of phimosis or meatal stenosis.

Laboratory Data

Urinalysis and culture, blood urea nitrogen (BUN), creatinine, and prostate-specific antigen (PSA) should be obtained. Urinalysis may suggest other possible causes for a man presenting with LUTS. Measurement of renal function (BUN and creatinine) may alert one to the severity of the obstruction. PSA determinations can help diagnose unsuspected prostate cancer (see Chapters 3 and 22) and give an estimate of prostate volume. Patients with a PSA of more than 1.6 ng/mL are at increased risk of urinary retention.

Uroflow/Postvoid Residual Urine

Measurement of the urine flow rate is the single best noninvasive method of estimating the degree of outlet obstruction. Peak flow rates of less than 15 mL/second (assuming a voided volume of >150 mL) are strong evidence of significant outflow obstruction. Measurement of postvoid residual urine (PVR), generally by noninvasive transabdominal ultrasound, can help identify patients who will respond to watchful waiting, medical, or surgical therapy. Patients with very reduced urinary flow rates (<10 mL/second) and postvoid residuals of more than 200 mL are at increased risk of urinary retention. More extensive urodynamic studies are generally not indicated in the routine workup of BPH.

Intravenous Urogram

Although not routinely indicated, an intravenous urogram (IVU) provides information about the upper tracts as well as the degree of residual urine. J-hooking of the lower ureters or elevation of the bladder base suggests marked intravesical prostatic enlargement. An IVU as routine screening for males with BPH has a low yield of incidental pathology (15%) and should be obtained only when otherwise indicated.

Cystourethroscopy

Cystourethroscopy is the only direct method of evaluating prostatic obstruction. The degree of lateral and median enlargement can be estimated. Inspect bladder for trabeculation, cellules, and diverticula. Examine bladder neck for contracture, bar formation, or a prominent median lobe. Estimate length of the posterior urethra and perform a water test for occlusion. Other pathologic causes such as bladder tumor or stones can be excluded. Cystoscopy can be performed in the office or just before prostatectomy, depending on the degree of uncertainty of the diagnosis.

TREATMENT

Treatment options for BPH continue to increase yearly. Transurethral resection of the prostate (TURP) is still the gold standard for severely symptomatic (IPSS >20) and obstructive BPH; however, many less invasive options have become popular. Most of these methods use different techniques, which range from lasers, radiofrequency, and microwaves, to heat the prostate to cause vaporization or coagulation necrosis. Medical management, primarily using α-blocker therapy or 5-α reductase medications, is the first line of treatment for patients with moderately symptomatic BPH (IPSS 9–19). Watchful waiting is appropriate for men with uncomplicated non-bothersome BPH.

Medical Therapy

■ $\alpha\text{-}_1$-Blockers

$\alpha\text{-}_1$-Adrenergic blocking agents are the most effective agents for relieving the IPSS symptoms of BPH. Tamsulosin (Flomax) is an antagonist of α_{1A}-subtype adrenergic receptors in the prostate and has been effectively used to relax prostatic smooth muscle fibers and decrease bladder outlet resistance. Terazosin and doxazosin appear to be as effective at relieving symptomatic BPH but have higher incidences of side effects (e.g., tiredness, dizziness, headache, and postural hypotension). A new $\alpha\text{-}_1$-blocker, alfzosin (Uroxatral), has a favorable pharmacokinetic profile which appears to minimize the typical side effects of this class of agents. Generally, α-blockers have been shown to increase peak urine flow rate and improve symptom scores (IPSS ~ 2 points) in about 60%.

■ 5-α -Reductase Inhibitor

5-α-Reductase inhibitors, such as dutasteride (Avodart) and finasteride (Proscar), are used to block intracellular conversion of testosterone to DHT. This approach attempts to shrink hyperplastic glands and reduce further progression of BPH. 5-α-Reductase inhibitors have been most effective in reducing the incidence of acute urinary retention in males with very large prostates (>50 mL) and improve IPSS approximately 1 to 2 points.

Combination Medical Therapy

Combining α-blocker therapy with a 5-α reductase inhibitor has been shown in a 5-year long-term therapy study (MTOPS) to be superior to either agent alone at preventing progression of LUTS and BPH; however, cost-effectiveness issues have been raised.

Surgical Therapy

Transurethral Resection of Prostate

Surgery is the gold standard for the treatment of BPH and produces the best improvements in symptoms and urine flow rates. TURP is the preferred method for all but the largest prostates that can be shelled out by open prostatectomy. In any simple prostatectomy, either TURP or open, the outer prostate gland is left in the surgical capsule. These patients are still at risk for developing prostate cancer. (Note there is a 10% incidence of unsuspected prostate cancer found in tissue removed for benign disease.) Approximately 70% of patients with secondary irritative symptoms (e.g., frequency, urgency, and nocturia) can be expected to have relief of these symptoms within 6 months of a TURP. The remaining 30% with persistent symptoms may require anticholinergic agents to control detrusor instability.

Indications for Surgery

- Urinary retention
- Hydronephrosis (with or without impaired renal function)
- Recurrent urinary tract infections (secondary to residual urine)
- Bladder stone (secondary to residual urine)
- Severe obstructive symptoms (with or without bladder instability)

Miscellaneous

Intraurethral Stents

Placement of metal self-retaining intraurethral stents may be effective in relieving urinary retention in patients who are not candidates for surgical management; however, complications of migration, encrustation, and discomfort limit their use.

■ Electrovaporization

Electrovaporization is a modification of the standard TURP using a metal roller with the diathermy set to a high current causing direct vaporization of the prostate with less hemorrhage. Long-term efficacy is unproved.

■ Laser Prostatectomy

Laser ablation of BPH using a neodynium:yttrium-aluminum-garnet (YAG) laser causes both vaporization and coagulation necrosis of the prostate by the high temperatures produced. However, these high temperatures can also cause postoperative pain and difficulty voiding for prolonged periods. Long-term outcome studies are still pending.

■ Hyperthermia

Other forms of hyperthermia have used radiofrequency energy such as in transurethral needle ablation (TUNA) and microwave energy in transurethral microwave thermotherapy (TUMT). These methods attempt to spare the urethra, thus minimizing side effects. However, a period requiring catheterization after these procedures is not uncommon, and further long-term outcome data will be necessary to fully evaluate their efficacy. Serious thermal injury complications have been reported.

Urinary Calculi

STONE FORMATION

The genesis of urinary stones requires both crystal formation and aggregation. Crystal formation occurs when concentrations of the stone components reach supersaturation within the urine at a specific temperature and pH. Intermittent supersaturation occurs frequently, for example, after meals or during periods of dehydration. These crystals must then aggregate to form stones and be retained within the kidney. Normal urine contains inhibitors of crystal formation and aggregation. Citrate and magnesium are inhibitors of crystal formation. Tamm-Horsfall protein and nephrocalcin are potent inhibitors of crystal aggregation.

TYPES AND CAUSES OF STONES

Calcium Stones (75%)

Calcium oxalate, as either a monohydrate or dihydrate (less dense), is a major component of most urinary stones. Calcium phosphate (apatite) is the second most common component of stones and is usually found in association with calcium oxalate. Both are highly insoluble salts in urine. Factors that are significant in calcium stone formation are discussed later. Hypercalciuria is the direct antecedent of most calcium stones.

■ Causes of Hypercalciuria

- *Increased intestinal absorption*—the mechanism of excessive intestinal calcium absorption that occurs in patients with idiopathic hypercalciuria is unknown; however, it is believed to be the most common etiology, accounting for approximately 50% of cases. Serum calcium is usually normal in the idiopathic group. Excessive vitamin D intake will also produce increased intestinal absorption resulting in hypercalcemia and hypercalciuria.

- *Decreased renal reabsorption*—the second major cause of idiopathic hypercalciuria is thought to be a "renal leak" mechanism. The loss of calcium in the urine leads to increased parathyroid hormone (PTH), which in turn causes elevated 1,25-vitamin D_3 and increased intestinal absorption to maintain normal serum levels of calcium.
- *Increased bone resorption*—the most common etiology of increased bone resorption is hyperparathyroidism; however, it accounts for less than 5% of stone patients. Parathyroid hyperplasia or adenomas secrete excessive amounts of PTH. PTH causes (a) increased calcium reabsorption in the proximal convoluted tubule, (b) increased 1,25-vitamin D_3, and (c) increased bone demineralization and calcium release from bone. Patients will have both elevated PTH and serum calcium levels. Other less frequent causes of resorptive hypercalciuria include chronic immobilization, metastatic cancer to bone, multiple myeloma, and vitamin D intoxication.

■ Differentiation of Hypercalciuric States

Type of Hypercalciuria	Serum Ca^{2+}	Urine Ca^{2+}	Serum PTH
Absorptive	Normal	Normal	Normal or increased
Renal	Normal	Increased	Increased
Idiopathic	Normal	Increased	Normal
Resorptive	Increased	Increased	Increased or normal

■ Hyperoxaluria

Oxalate is a major component of most calcium stones and has an effect on crystallization that is ten times greater than that of calcium. Eighty percent of urinary oxalate comes from endogenous production in the liver (40% from ascorbic acid, 40% from glycine) and 20% from dietary sources. Foods high in oxalate are tea, coffee, beer, rhubarb, cocoa, spinach, and other green leafy vegetables. The primary site of oxalate absorption is the distal bowel (colon). Patients with small bowel resection (or bypass) or inflammatory bowel disease can have increased oxalate absorption.

■ Hyperuricosuria

Uric acid promotes calcium oxalate crystal formation. Hyperuricosuria with normal urine pH (>5.5) is frequently associated with calcium stones.

■ Hypocitraturia

Citrate in the urine has an inhibitory effect on stone formation by binding with calcium in the urine and thereby decreasing calcium oxalate and calcium phosphate crystal formation. A low urinary citrate level is associated with calcium nephrolithiasis in 20% to 60% of patients with stone formation. Conditions that can result in hypocitraturia are renal tubular acidosis (RTA), strenuous exercise, enteric hyperoxaluria, and diets high in animal protein.

■ Type I (Distal) Renal Tubular Acidosis

Type I RTA is caused by an inability of the distal nephron to establish and maintain a hydrogen ion gradient between the tubular fluid and the blood (see Chapter 28). It causes primarily calcium phosphate stone formation in up to 70% of adults with the disorder because of hypocitraturia and hypercalciuria. The diagnosis of Type I RTA is made by finding hypokalemia, hyperchloremia, metabolic acidosis, and a urine pH of 5.5 or higher. Giving potassium citrate corrects the hypocitraturia, hypokalemia, and metabolic acidosis.

Infection Stones (Struvite) (15%)

Magnesium ammonium phosphate ($MgNH_4PO_4$-$6H_2O$) or "triple phosphate" stones occur in the setting of persistently high urinary pH caused by urea-splitting bacteria, resulting in high ammonia production. Alkaline pH higher than 7.2 markedly reduces the solubility of magnesium ammonium phosphate in urine, resulting in its precipitation. The major urea-splitting organisms include *Proteus* species, *Pseudomonas*, and *Klebsiella*. Neurogenic bladder and foreign bodies in the urinary tract (e.g., catheters and sutures—even chromic catgut) have a high association with formation of struvite calculi. Struvite stones have been shown to contain numerous infective bacteria within their structure where antibiotics cannot penetrate; therefore, they must be removed if infection is to be cured. Prophylaxis against recurring magnesium ammonium phosphate stones requires maintenance of sterile urine (long-term suppressive antibiotics), high urine volumes, and decreased urinary phosphate levels (limit dietary phosphate ingestion and intestinal absorption by administering phosphate-binding aluminum hydroxide gels). Struvite calculi account for most staghorn stones.

Uric Acid Stones (5%–10%)

Uric acid is a product of purine metabolism and is excreted in the urine. Stones form in the setting of low urine volume, low pH (acid urine), and high levels of urinary uric acid (hyperuricosuria). They are the only radiolucent urinary calculi. Uric acid stone formers can be categorized into two major groups: those with high blood levels of uric acid and those with normal levels.

■ Hyperuricosuria without Hyperuricemia

Causes of isolated uric acid stones include a consistently abnormal low pH (e.g., patients with chronic diarrheal states or those taking acidifying medications), excessive water loss (especially from the gastrointestinal tract), uricosuric drugs (e.g., salicylates and thiazides), and high-protein diets. Management of these patients consists of increasing urinary volume to 2 L/day (or 1 L urine output for every 300 mg uric acid in a 24-hour urine collection), limiting dietary proteins to less than 90 g/day, and alkalinizing urine (to a level between pH 6.5 and 7.0).

■ Hyperuricosuria with Hyperuricemia

Elevated serum uric acid levels can be caused by gout, myeloproliferative disorders (acute leukemia), or neoplastic disease and the Lesch-Nyhan syndrome (an inborn error of metabolism owing to a deficiency of the enzyme hypoxanthine-guanine phosphoribosyltransferase). These patients will usually require treatment with allopurinol 300 mg/day, in addition to the previous measures.

Cystine Stones (1%)

Cystinuria is the result of an inherited autosomal recessive defect in the renal tubular reabsorption of four amino acids: cystine, ornithine, lysine, and arginine (mnemonic COLA). Normal urinary cystine levels are less than 100 mg per 24 hours; however, homozygous cystinurics excrete in excess of 600 mg/day. Ask about a family history of stone disease or recurrent stones and look for the characteristic hexagonal cystine crystals or a positive cyanide nitroprusside test in the urine. Stones may also occur in heterozygous cystinurics that excrete less than 300 mg/day. Cystine stones occur in acid urine. Management of cystinuria consists of increasing urinary volume to 3 to 4 L/day (or >1 L urine output for every 300 mg cystine in a 24-hour urine collection) and urinary alkalinization to pH greater than 7.0. In resistant cases, D-penicillamine (250 mg q6h) or α-mercaptopropionylglycine (MPG) (250 mg q6h) can be used to enhance cystine solubility in urine. Cystine stones can occasionally form staghorns.

MANAGEMENT OF UROLITHIASIS

Management of urolithiasis has undergone a major revolution since the development of extracorporeal shock wave lithotripsy (ESWL) and advances in endoscopic equipment. The combination of ESWL and endourologic technology has almost eliminated major open stone surgery. Approximately 50% of symptomatic stones will require surgical intervention, and 50% can be expected to pass spontaneously. Stones of less than 5 mm in diameter should generally be given 4 to 8 weeks to pass on their own if definitive indications for removal do not exist. Stones of greater than 10 mm are unlikely to pass, and interventional therapy should be planned.

Most Common Sites for Hang-Up of Ureteral Stones

- Ureteropelvic junction
- Pelvic brim where ureter crosses iliac vessels
- Just outside bladder at base of broad ligament in females or where vas deferens crosses ureter in males
- Ureterovesical junction in intramural ureter

Indications for Early Intervention

- High-grade urinary obstruction
- Persistent infection despite antibiotics
- Uncontrollable pain
- Impairment of renal function

Stone Dissolution

Unfortunately, most stones (i.e., calcium stones) cannot be dissolved. Uric acid or cystine stones can frequently be dissolved by alkalinization of the urine. If there is significant ureteral obstruction, a stent should be placed. Oral alkalinization (sodium bicarbonate or potassium citrate) may require several weeks. Titrate urine pH with Nitrazine paper. Direct irrigation of the stone via percutaneous or retrograde catheters with an alkaline solution is occasionally successful. Hyperuricosuria can be managed by a low-purine diet or allopurinol if urine uric acid levels exceed 1,200 mg/day. A diet low in methionine can help lower urinary cystine levels. Dissolution therapy should be given

1 month before deeming it a failure. Failure to dissolve the stones will require surgical intervention.

■ Dissolution of Uric Acid Stones

- Increase urine volume to at least 2 L/day.
- Titrate urine pH to 6.5 to 7.0 with potassium citrate [10–20 mEq orally (PO) twice a day (bid) to four times a day (qid)].
- Adopt low-purine diet (decrease red meats).
- Use allopurinol 300 mg/day if patient is unresponsive to low-purine diet or if urine uric acid is greater than 1,200 mg/day.

■ Dissolution of Cystine Stones

- Alkalinize urine to pH greater than 7.0 with potassium citrate.
- Increase fluid intake to greater than 4 L/day.
- Restrict foods high in methionine such as meat and dairy products.
- Administer D-penicillamine or α-MPG if unresponsive.

Surgical Management

■ Treatment Modalities

Extracorporeal shock wave lithotripsy. ESWL uses shock waves produced by electrical spark gap or electromagnetic or piezo-electric energy sources. The shock wave is then transmitted through a water medium to the patient. The stone is positioned at the second focal point of the shock wave by a three-dimensional fluoroscopic scanning system or by ultrasound imaging. The similar impedance of the human body and water allows efficient energy transfer to the stone, resulting in fragmentation (note that cystine stones respond poorly to ESWL).

Endourology. Stone extraction can often be performed by manually grasping the stone with special forceps or by trapping the stone within one of several instruments that look like a wire basket and then removing the stone. Stones too large to be directly removed endoscopically must first be fragmented into smaller pieces using laser, electrohydraulic, or ultrasound techniques. Manually crushing the stone is also an option under certain circumstances. Stones can be approached endoscopically in a retrograde fashion through the urethra and ureter or in an anterograde fashion with a percutaneous nephrostomy.

Open surgery. Open surgery for stones such as a pyelolithotomy, nephrolithotomy, or ureterolithotomy is rarely necessary if access to ESWL and endourologic technology is available.

■ Treatment by Stone Location

Kidney. ESWL and/or endourologic stone fragmentation via a nephrostomy tract or a retrograde approach is the treatment of choice. Open surgical removal is occasionally necessary for complicated cases or large staghorn calculi.

Ureter. Upper ureteral stones above the iliac crest can generally be treated with primary ESWL. Lower ureteral stones can be repositioned endoscopically to above the iliac crest and then treated with ESWL. Primary ureteroscopic extraction with or without laser lithotripsy is effective for lower ureteral stones and some upper ureteral stones.

Bladder and urethra. Vesical calculi can generally be removed cystoscopically with laser or electrohydraulic lithotripsy. Urethral stones can usually be grasped with forceps and removed or pushed back into the bladder with or without the use of laser lithotripsy. Open cystolithotomy is occasionally necessary.

WORKUP OF STONE-FORMING PATIENTS

Initial evaluation and acute management of the stone patient are covered in the section on management of urolithiasis and in Chapter 6. A brief guide follows to help approach stone-forming patients after acute therapy has been rendered and the stone removed. Diagnosing the underlying etiology of a patient's stone disease is essential if future stone recurrences are to be avoided. Approximately 15% of patients will have a recurrence within 1 year and nearly 50% within 5 years. Patients with their first stone will generally be given a limited screen looking for significant metabolic risk factors. Patients with recurrent stones or with abnormalities on their first stone screen should undergo a more extensive workup.

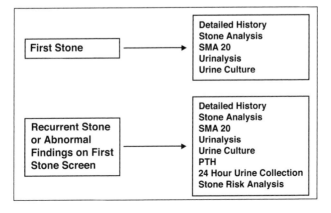

History

A detailed history is essential. Question about infections, medications (including herbal supplements), diet (including vitamins), bowel disease or surgery, gout, renal disease, bone or parathyroid disease, and any family history of stone disease. Particular attention should be paid to fluid intake and any dietary indiscretions. A dietary diary for 1 week is helpful.

Metabolic Workup

■ Stone Analysis

Results of a stone chemical analysis are invaluable in guiding management. Every effort should be made to retrieve the stone.

■ Blood Tests

SMA-20 will include electrolytes, serum calcium, uric acid, and phosphorus. A PTH level should be obtained.

■ Urine Assessment

- Urinalysis (include pH and check for crystals) and urine culture should be obtained.
- A cyanide nitroprusside test of the urine can be used to screen for suspected cystinuria.
- A 24-hour urine collection on a random diet should be performed for calcium, phosphorus, magnesium, oxalate, uric acid, citrate, total volume, and creatinine and then repeated on a restricted diet (avoid meat and restrict sodium, oxalate, and calcium).

STONE PREVENTION

Prevention of recurrent stones is an important aspect of the overall care of the stone-forming patient. High fluid intake with the goal of more than 2-L urine output per day is the single most important modification that can be recommended for all stone-forming patients. All patients should also be encouraged to eliminate any dietary excesses (especially protein and phosphates), and moderate sodium restriction is beneficial for patients with hypercalciuria. Potassium citrate has become increasingly important in the management of all stone-forming patients except infection stones.

Potassium citrate alkalinizes the urine for patients with uric acid or cystine stones and supplements urinary citrate levels and its inhibitory effect on calcium stone formation. Patients with hyperuricemia should be put on a low-protein diet (<90 g/day) and allopurinol if urine uric acid levels exceed 1,200 mg/day or serum uric acid levels are abnormal.

Urinary alkalinization is usually accomplished by giving oral potassium citrate and titrating the dose to the appropriate urine pH monitored with Nitrazine paper. The suggested dosages of potassium citrate are only starting points and should be adjusted as needed to accomplish the goal.

Calcium Stone–Forming Patients

The mainstay in preventing recurrent calcium oxalate or calcium phosphate stones is to increase fluid intake and supplement with potassium citrate. The addition of a thiazide diuretic is indicated for high urinary calcium levels and allopurinol for high urinary uric acid levels (>1,200 mg/day). Hyperuricosuria has been shown to promote calcium oxalate stone formation. Moderate sodium restriction is also beneficial to patients with hypercalciuria, especially if they are taking a thiazide diuretic.

Dietary calcium restriction, once a mainstay of preventing calcium nephrolithiasis, has come into question. Recent studies have reported that a *higher* intake of dietary calcium was strongly associated with a *decreased* risk of kidney stones. Dietary calcium restriction is thus inappropriate. However, dietary calcium supplementation has not been shown to be protective against calcium stones.

■ Normocalciuria (and Normocalcemia)

Increase fluid (>2 L/day) and prescribe potassium citrate (Urocit-K 20 mEq PO bid).

■ Hypercalciuria (and Normocalcemia)

Increase fluid (>3 L/day) and prescribe potassium citrate (Urocit-K 20 mEq PO bid) and thiazide diuretic (HCTZ 25 mg PO bid).

■ Hypercalcemia

The patient should be worked up for hyperparathyroidism.

▨ Hyperuricosuria

Increase fluid (>3 L/day) and prescribe potassium citrate (Urocit-K 20 mEq PO bid) and allopurinol [Zyloprim 300 mg PO daily (qd)] if urine uric acid levels exceed 1,200 mg/day.

▨ Hyperuricemia

Increase fluid (>3 L/day) and prescribe potassium citrate (Urocit-K 20 mEq PO bid) and allopurinol (Zyloprim 300 mg PO qd).

▨ Hyperoxaluria

Patients with increased oxalate absorption in the gut are treated as for other findings and dietary oxalate restriction. In addition, calcium carbonate (1–2 g with each meal) or cholestyramine will inhibit oxalate absorption.

▨ Type I (Distal) Renal Tubular Acidosis

Type I RTA causes primarily calcium phosphate stone formation because of hypocitraturia and hypercalciuria. Giving potassium citrate corrects both hypocitraturia and metabolic acidosis.

Struvite Stone Formers

Prevention of recurrent magnesium ammonium phosphate stones requires complete surgical removal of any stone, alleviation of any obstruction, and maintenance of sterile urine. Occasionally acetohydroxamic acid (250 mg PO q8h), a reversible inhibitor of urease, may be used to help prevent crystallization of struvite.

Uric Acid Stone Formers

Patients with hyperuricemia should be managed with increased fluid (>3 L/day), potassium citrate (Urocit-K 20 mEq PO bid), and allopurinol (Zyloprim 300 mg PO qd). Patients with hyperuricosuria and normal serum uric acid levels should be treated with allopurinol if urinary uric acid levels exceed 1,200 mg/day. All patients who form uric acid stones should have their urine alkalinized to pH 6.5 to 7.0. It should not be raised above 7.0. Titrate urine pH with Nitrazine paper. Allopurinol inhibits xanthine oxidase and decreases the production of uric acid. It is dosed at either 300 mg PO qd or 100 mg PO tid.

Cystine Stone Formers

Restrict foods high in methionine such as meat and dairy products. Fluid intake should be increased (>3 L/day) and the urine should be alkalinized with potassium citrate (Urocit-K 20 mEq PO bid). A urine pH of higher than 7.0 is the goal. If alkalinization fails, then D-penicillamine and α-MPG are used to complex with cystine and form soluble compounds.

NEUROPHYSIOLOGY OF VOIDING

The act of micturition is a complex reflex function under voluntary control. The following diagram gives a simplified way of understanding the general neurologic innervation of the bladder and sphincter mechanisms. The coordination of the micturition reflex (i.e., detrusor contraction with sphincter relaxation) is controlled by the brainstem (pontine) micturition center via the long spinal (loop II) pathways to the sacral cord (S2, S3, S4). This in turn is under voluntary control by suprapontine higher functions via loop I.

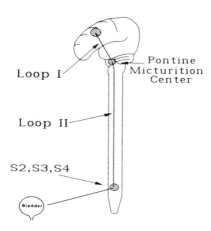

Detrusor hyperreflexia with a coordinated external sphincter is caused by suprapontine lesions involving loop I (e.g., stroke, Parkinson's disease, and tumors) as well as nonneurologic local causes (e.g., infection, outlet obstruction, tumor, stone, foreign body).

Detrusor hyperreflexia with external sphincter dyssynergia is generally caused by suprasacral spinal lesions involving loop II (e.g., tumor, multiple sclerosis, myelodysplasia, and spinal arteriovenous malformations).

Detrusor areflexia can result from interruption of sacral reflex arcs (e.g., diabetic neuropathy, multiple sclerosis, herniated disks, and spinal cord tumors), as well as direct myogenic causes (e.g., prolonged urinary retention). Areflexia also occurs during the period of spinal shock after suprasacral spinal cord injury.

CLASSIFICATIONS OF DYSFUNCTIONAL VOIDING

Many classification systems have been promoted for categorizing voiding disorders based on neuroanatomic, urodynamic, or functional criteria. The Wein classification system is a beautifully simplistic functional categorization based on the failure of the bladder to store or empty. It serves most clinical voiding disorders well, whether of neurogenic or nonneurogenic origin, and helps guide one toward the correct treatment options.

Functional Classification of Voiding Disorders

Failure to Store	Failure to Empty
• Because of the bladder	• Because of the bladder
• Because of the outlet	• Because of the outlet

Failures to store because of the bladder simply include involuntary bladder contractions, low compliance, and hypersensitivity, whereas outlet problems are simply due to inadequate outlet resistance. Failures to empty because of the bladder are a result of poor or no bladder contractility, whereas outlet problems are from mechanical [e.g., benign prostatic hyperplasia (BPH), stricture] or functional (dyssynergia) obstruction. Combination deficits can also occur as in spinal cord injury (detrusor hyperreflexia and sphincter dyssynergia).

Detrusor hyperreflexia refers to involuntary bladder contractions on urodynamic studies caused by a neurologic disorder, whereas involuntary contractions without a neurologic cause are termed detrusor instability. More popular today is the general term overactive bladder, which refers to the symptoms of frequency and urgency without urodynamic confirmation of detrusor hyperreflexia or instability.

URODYNAMICS

Urodynamics is the study of lower urinary tract physiology. It is a complex field that includes uroflowmetry, cystometry, urethral pressure profilometry, and electromyography. Even a brief overview of all these areas is beyond the scope of this manual.

Only basic uroflowmetry and cystometry are covered because they are generally all that are required for most clinical urodynamic workups. Remember that a detailed history is the foundation of any evaluation of a voiding disorder.

Urinary Flow Rate/Residual Urine

The combination of a uroflow followed by determination of the residual urine is the most useful test in the study of any voiding disorder. Urinary flow rate is best recorded on an electronic flowmeter, which plots the flow pattern in a graphic representation of instantaneous flow rate versus voiding time.

Peak uroflow rate is the only objective measure of functional bladder outlet obstruction, and it is directly dependent on the volume voided. Peak flows measured when the voided volume was less than 150 mL should be disregarded.

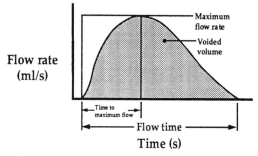

Use of this flow nomogram allows a more accurate determination of outflow resistance by removing the effect of intravesical volume on flow rate. Peak flow rates more than two standard deviations below the mean are highly suggestive of outflow obstruction.

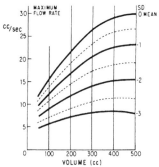

Cystometry

Cystometry is generally used to evaluate bladder filling and storage. A cystometrogram is a pressure/volume curve obtained by filling the bladder with a fluid (either water or carbon dioxide) at a constant infusion rate while monitoring changes in intravesical pressure. The patient is asked to inhibit any urge to void during the study. Any detrusor contractions greater than 15 cmH$_2$O are considered abnormal or uninhibited contractions. A voiding phase cystometrogram may be obtained at the end of the study when the patient has a strong urge to void by asking him or her to voluntarily urinate around the catheter.

Data to be noted during the cystometrogram include the following:
1. Volume at first sensation of filling (proprioception)
2. Volume at sensation of fullness
3. Volume at desire to void
4. Occurrence of a voluntary detrusor contraction when asked to void
5. Ability to inhibit a voluntary detrusor contraction

NORMAL CYSTOMETROGRAM

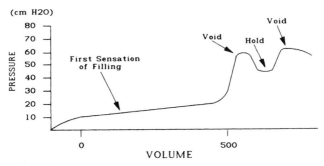

■ **Normal Cystometrogram**

A normal cystometrogram should demonstrate a first sensation of filling at 100 to 200 mL, normal accommodation with continued filling and good compliance (i.e., <10 cmH$_2$O change in intravesical pressure), and a sensation of fullness and desire to urinate at 350 to 450 mL. Asking the patient to produce a voluntary detrusor contraction at the end of the study is often unsuccessful because of the patient's inability to properly relax in the test setting. Normal sensation and compliance with an absence of uninhibited contractions are all that are needed to consider the study normal.

UROPHARMACOLOGY

Overview

Bladder contraction is mediated by stimulation of the parasympathetic nervous system and release of acetylcholine. Cholinergic muscarinic receptors are located in the dome of the bladder. Five muscarinic receptor subtypes (M1–M5) have been identified. M3 receptors appear to be primary in detrusor contraction, perhaps with assistance for M2 receptors.

α-Adrenergic receptors in the bladder neck and urethra moderate smooth muscle contraction and increase outlet resistance on stimulation by the sympathetic nervous system. β-Adrenergic receptors in the dome of the bladder facilitate accommodation during filling by causing smooth muscle relaxation in the bladder.

Pharmacotherapy for voiding disorders has been disappointingly ineffective on the whole. Despite the pharmacologic effectiveness of certain drugs, clinical improvement is impeded by a lack of specificity of the agent and untoward side effects on other organ systems with similar receptors at pharmacologic doses.

Drugs to Facilitate Storage

▓ Decrease Bladder Contractility

- Propantheline (Pro-Banthine) is an anticholinergic that blocks bladder contraction by competitive blockade at receptors of parasympathetic postganglionic nerve endings. It is variably effective in patients with uninhibited hyperreflexic neurogenic bladders. Side effects include dry mouth, visual disturbances, and constipation [dosage: 15 mg orally (PO) three times a day (tid)/four times a day (qid)].
- Oxybutynin (Ditropan) has a direct antispasmodic effect on smooth muscle and blocks cholinergic receptors. It has variable clinical effectiveness in patients with uninhibited bladder contractions (dosage: 5 mg PO tid/qid). Oxybutynin extended release (Ditropan XL) is dosed once a day and has fewer side effects [dosage: 5–10 mg PO daily (qd)]. Oxybutynin transdermal patch (Oxytrol) is a form of immediate release oxybutynin (dosage: 3.9 mg patch twice per week).
- Tolterodine tartrate (Detrol) is a competitive muscarinic receptor antagonist indicated for treatment of bladder overactivity [dosage: 2 mg PO twice a day (bid)]. An extended release

formulation of tolterodine (Detrol LA) is a once-daily formulation (dosage: 4 mg PO qd).

- Flavoxate (Urispas) has anticholinergic, local, anesthetic, and analgesic properties and may also have a direct relaxant effect on smooth muscle. Flavoxate has been used to reduce irritative voiding symptoms and suprapubic pain (dosage: 100–200 mg PO tid/qid).
- Trospium (Sanctura) is a balanced M3/M2 selective anticholinergic (dosage: 20 mg PO bid).
- Darifenacin (Enablex) is an M3 selective anticholinergic (dosage: 7.5–15 mg PO qd).
- Solifenacin (VESIcare) is an antimuscarinic with smooth muscle relaxing properties (dosage: 5–10 mg PO qd).
- Imipramine (Tofranil) has been shown to be clinically effective in facilitating urine storage; however, its mechanism of action is unclear. Peripheral anticholinergic and sympathomimetic actions have been noted in addition to a direct smooth muscle relaxation. Thus, it decreases bladder contractility and increases outlet resistance. It is effective for controlling bedwetting in children (dosage: 25 mg PO tid/qid).
- Hyoscyamine sulfate (Levsin) is one of the principal anticholinergic/antispasmodic components of belladonna alkaloids. Hyoscyamine has been effective in the treatment of spastic neurogenic bladders [dosage: 1–2 tablets (0.125 mg) PO/sublingual (SL) q4h]. Extended release hyoscyamine (Levbid) affords better dosing (dosage: 1 tablet PO bid).
- Dicyclomine (Bentyl) has direct smooth muscle relaxant and anticholinergic effects primarily indicated for irritable bowel syndrome (dosage: 20 mg PO tid).

■ Increase Outlet Resistance

- Ephedrine is an α-adrenergic agonist that causes contraction of smooth muscle of the bladder outlet and urethral sphincter. Dosage is 25 to 50 mg PO qid.
- Phenylpropanolamine (Ornade) is also an α-adrenergic agonist and thus causes increased bladder outlet resistance secondary to smooth muscle contraction (dosage: 50 mg PO bid).
- Estrogens are believed to increase outlet resistance in females with stress incontinence by increasing α-adrenergic receptor sensitivity and improving the mucosal seal of the urethral wall (dosage: Estrace vaginal cream 1/2 g Monday, Wednesday, Friday).

Drugs to Facilitate Emptying

▦ Increase Bladder Contractility

- Bethanechol chloride (Urecholine) is a cholinergic agonist that acts at the postganglionic parasympathetic effector cells to enhance contraction of smooth muscle. Oral Urecholine is largely ineffective clinically.

▦ Decrease Outlet Resistance

- Phenoxybenzamine (Dibenzyline) is an α-adrenergic blocking agent that has been shown to be effective in blocking hyperactivity of the bladder outlet smooth muscle sphincter. However, it has negative systemic effects (orthostatic hypotension), and it has been shown to have in vitro mutagenic activity. These factors have significantly curtailed its use.
- Prazosin (Minipress) is also an α-adrenergic blocking agent that has been used to inhibit bladder neck contractility. Its negative effects include postural hypotension, reflex tachycardia, nasal congestion, inhibition of seminal emission, and retrograde ejaculation. Initial dosage is 1 mg bid or tid.
- Terazosin (Hytrin) is a selective α_1-blocking agent that has been used to relax smooth muscle fibers of the prostate and bladder neck. It requires only once a day dosing starting at 1 mg/day initially. Dosages of 2 to 10 mg/day may be necessary. Dose must be titrated.
- Doxazosin (Cardura) is another selective α_1-blocking agent with activity and side effects similar to those of terazosin (dosage: 2–8 mg PO qd). Dose must be titrated.
- Tamsulosin (Flomax) is a highly selective antagonist of the α_{1a}-subtype adrenoceptors. It promotes smooth muscle relaxation in the bladder neck and prostatic urethra. Dose titration is unnecessary (dosage: 0.4 mg PO qd).
- Alfuzosin (Uroxatral) is an extended release selective antagonist of α_1-adrenoceptors (dosage: 10 mg PO qd).
- Diazepam (Valium) has striated muscle relaxant ability but has had only limited success in treating external sphincter dyssynergia at tolerable dosages.
- Dantrolene (Dantrium) also has striated muscle relaxant effects but limited success in treating external sphincter dyssynergia at tolerable dosages. It has a significant risk of producing fatal hepatotoxicity and should, therefore, be avoided.
- Baclofen (Lioresal) is a polysynaptic inhibitor of both the bladder and outlet with muscle relaxant and antispasmodic activity. It has some limited usefulness in treating external sphincter dyssynergia.

MANAGEMENT

Therapy for voiding disorders consists of surgical, pharmacologic, or mechanical interventions. After determining whether the patient has primarily a storage or an emptying disorder, the following brief lists can help guide therapy.

To Promote Storage

■ Decrease Bladder Contractility

- Removal of local irritative factors (treat infection or tumors and remove stones or foreign bodies)
- Pharmacotherapy (oxybutynin, tolterodine, solifenacin, trospium, darifenacin)
- Surgery: bladder denervation (cystolysis) and augmentation cystoplasty

■ Increase Outlet Resistance

- Pharmacotherapy (ephedrine, imipramine, phenylpropanolamine)
- Biofeedback or electrical stimulation
- Surgery (bladder neck sling, collagen injection, artificial sphincters)

■ Bypass Problem

- Condom catheter, Foley catheter, or urinary diversion

Drug Therapy for Voiding Disorders

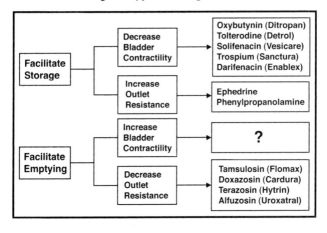

To Promote Emptying

▦ Increase Bladder Contractility

- No clinically effective therapy

▦ Decrease Outlet Resistance

- Pharmacotherapy (terazosin, doxazosin, tamsulosin, alfuzosin, diazepam, baclofen)
- Surgery: transurethral resection of the prostate, incision of strictures, urethral dilatation, urethroplasty, Y-V plasty of bladder neck, external sphincterotomy

▦ Bypass Problem

- External bladder compression (Crede's method)
- Catheterization: intermittent or continuous
- Surgery: urinary diversion

SPECIFIC GUIDELINES

Failure to Store

▦ Because of the Bladder

1. *Infection.* The local irritative effects of cystitis or prostatitis can produce significant frequency and urgency. Treat with appropriate antibiotic therapy.
2. *Outlet obstruction.* Bladder outlet obstruction from BPH or strictures produces a primary disorder of failure to empty with a secondary disorder of failure to store (i.e., frequency, urgency, and nocturia) because of bladder instability. Correction of the primary disorder will usually result in resolution of the secondary bladder instability.
3. *Tumor.* A bladder tumor can cause significant local irritability manifested by frequency and urgency. Treat the tumor.
4. *Bladder stone.* A stone can cause a primary local irritative focus in the bladder that is often compounded by a secondary infection. Removal of the stone and eradication of infection should be effective.
5. *Poor compliance.* Decreased bladder compliance is usually secondary to inflammation, obstruction, or neurogenic causes. Elimination of the primary disorder is the goal. The small fibrotic contracted bladder may require augmentation cystoplasty or urinary diversion.
6. *Neurogenic hyperreflexia.* A hyperreflexic neurogenic bladder can be managed by pharmacotherapy (oxybutynin, tolterodine, solifenacin, darifenacin) or can be converted to a failure

to empty by augmentation cystoplasty and placed on clean intermittent catheterization (CIC).

▓ Because of the Outlet

1. *Sphincter incompetence.* Incompetent internal or external sphincter mechanisms can be managed with pharmacotherapy (ephedrine, imipramine, phenylpropanolamine) and surgical procedures (bladder neck sling, artificial sphincters). Failures must be consigned to condom catheters, Foley catheters, or urinary diversion.

Failure to Empty

▓ Because of the Bladder

- *Areflexia.* There is no effective means of increasing detrusor contractility. Patients are best managed with CIC, indwelling Foley catheter, or urinary diversion.

▓ Because of the Outlet

- *Outlet obstruction.* Mechanical outlet obstruction from BPH or strictures requires relief of the primary disorder (e.g., transurethral resection of the prostate, pharmacotherapy, or urethrotomy).
- *Sphincter dyssynergia.* Detrusor hyperreflexia with sphincter dyssynergia is a combined disorder of a failure to store and a failure to empty. The hyperactive uncoordinated external sphincter produces a functional outlet obstruction while the detrusor hyperreflexia results in small functional bladder capacities. These patients are best managed by first converting them to a primary disorder of emptying by pharmacotherapy, cystolysis, or bladder augmentation and then using CIC to empty the bladder.

Spinal Cord Injury

Injury to the spinal cord can result in various patterns of function based on the degree and level of the injury. Initial evaluation, including urodynamic testing and intravenous urography, should be conducted approximately 8 weeks after the injury. A period of spinal shock, usually lasting several days to weeks after the injury, can be expected. During this time, cord segments below the level of the injury will demonstrate decreased excitability. Detrusor areflexia with a continent internal urethral sphincter is the rule. Intermittent or chronic catheterization will be necessary. Recovery of reflex vesical activity with sphincter dyssynergia is the most common outcome in patients with suprasacral lesions. If intravesical pressures are elevated (>40 cm H_2O), upper tract damage can be expected if treatment is not undertaken. Lesions of the sacral cord or cauda equina usually result in detrusor areflexia with low bladder pressures and can be safely managed with intermittent catheterization.

■ Autonomic Dysreflexia

Autonomic dysreflexia is a syndrome characterized by a major sympathetic nervous response to afferent visceral stimulation in the spinal cord injury patient. Clinical manifestations include sweating, piloerection, a pounding headache, bradycardia, a widened pulse pressure, and a subjective sense of impending doom on the part of the patient. This can occur in response to stimulation of the bladder, urethra, or rectum in patients with cord lesions above T5, usually in the cervical region, and most frequently during the period from 3 to 8 months after injury. Acute bladder filling as occurs during cystoscopy or urodynamic testing can trigger an episode. Catheter drainage of the bladder can be used to minimize chronic autonomic dysreflexia.

Treatment

Treatment of an acute episode is with nifedipine (sublingual), hydralazine, or phentolamine and removal of the afferent stimulus (i.e., drain the bladder). Chlorpromazine (Thorazine), 25 mg IM q6h, can be used prophylactically in patients with potential for such a response during cystoscopy.

Prostate Cancer

Prostate cancer is the second most common cause of cancer deaths in men, with close to 35,000 deaths and more than 125,000 new cases per year in the United States. Blacks appear to have a 50% higher incidence and mortality. No clear etiologic factors have been identified, although a familial predisposition has been demonstrated, and an increased risk has been associated with cigarette smoking and a high-fat diet.

PATHOLOGY

Greater than 95% of prostate cancers are acinar adenocarcinomas. Other infrequent types include ductal carcinomas and carcinosarcomas.

Ductal Carcinomas

Accounting for less than 5% of prostate cancers, ductal carcinomas include transitional and squamous cell carcinomas, intraductal adenocarcinomas and mixed ductal carcinomas, and endometrioid carcinomas. Patients commonly have hematuria, positive urinary cytologies, and normal prostate-specific antigen (PSA). Treatment is cystoprostatectomy if localized to the prostate. Metastases are generally osteolytic rather than osteoblastic, and most do not respond to androgen withdrawal; however, if elements of acinar adenocarcinoma are present, hormonal therapy may be beneficial.

Carcinosarcomas

These uncommon tumors contain various mesenchymal elements and have a poor prognosis. (The remainder of this discussion will concern *only* acinar adenocarcinoma of the prostate.)

Adenocarcinoma of the Prostate

Adenocarcinomas of the prostate arise primarily in the peripheral zone (70%); however, 20% arise in the transition zone and about 5% in the central zone. Spread is by direct local extension and by lymphatic and vascular channels. Invasion of the capsule followed by extension to the seminal vesicles and bladder base indicates a more aggressive tumor. Ureteral obstruction occurs in 10% to 35% of patients with advanced disease. Direct extension to the rectum is rare. Lymphatic drainage is primarily to the obturator and hypogastric nodes. Osteoblastic bony metastasis is the most common location of distant spread, usually in the axial skeleton, such as the lumbar spine, proximal femur, pelvis, thoracic spine, ribs, sternum, and skull. Visceral metastases are commonest in the lung, liver, and adrenals.

GLEASON'S GRADING SYSTEM

Gleason's system uses five different histologic patterns (1–5) to characterize the degree of glandular differentiation under low-power magnification. It grades the two most representative areas of the tumor, called the primary and secondary grades, and adds those two values, giving a final Gleason score (also known as Gleason's sum or combined Gleason's grade) between 2 and 10. Cytologic features play no role in the grade of the tumor. A high Gleason score indicates increased dedifferentiation, increased risk of nodal metastases, and a more malignant potential. There is good correlation between Gleason's sum and prognosis. Interobserver and intraobserver reproducibility is generally within one Gleason's sum. The presence of Gleason's pattern 4 or Gleason's sum 7 or more is predictive of a poor prognosis.

TNM STAGING SYSTEM

The clinical stage is an assessment of the extent of tumor based primarily on the digital rectal examination (DRE), PSA, and Gleason's grade, in addition to any imaging modalities. The pathologic stage is based on histologic examination of the prostate and lymph nodes after surgical removal. The criteria most predictive of the prognosis are Gleason's grade and pathologic stage, including the surgical margin status, presence of extracapsular disease, seminal vesicle invasion, and involvement of pelvic lymph nodes.

Nomograms have been developed for the prediction of pathologic stage based on the clinical T stage, PSA level, and Gleason's score from needle biopsy specimens (Partin AW, et al. *JAMA* 1997;277:1445–1451). These tables have proved useful in counseling men with newly diagnosed prostate cancer about treatment alternatives.

Clinical Staging	
T1	Tumor not clinically apparent—nonpalpable
T1a	Incidental finding at TURP 5% or less of tissue resected
T1b	Incidental finding at TURP >5% of tissue resected
T1c	Needle biopsy finding—nonpalpable—elevated PSA only
T2	Palpable tumor confined within the prostate
T2a	Tumor involves one lobe
T2b	Tumor involves both lobes
T3	Tumor extends through prostatic capsule
T3a	Unilateral extracapsular extension
T3b	Bilateral extracapsular extension
T3c	Tumor invades seminal vesicle(s)
T4	Tumor invades adjacent structures (bladder, sphincter, rectum, etc.)

Pathologic Staging	
T2a	Organ confined—unilateral
T2b	Organ confined—bilateral
T3a	Unilateral extracapsular extension
T3b	Bilateral extracapsular extension
T3c	Seminal vesicle invasion
T4	Invasion of bladder or rectum

PSA, prostate-specific antigen; TURP, transurethral resection of the prostate.

PRESENTATION

Prostate cancer is a disease of the elderly, with 75% of patients diagnosed between age 60 and 85 years and a mean age at diagnosis of 72 years. Recent surveys report that an increasing percentage of patients are being diagnosed with earlier stage disease than in the past. The widespread use of the serum PSA test has been important in early diagnosis.

Most patients are asymptomatic at the time of diagnosis. Prostate cancer is most commonly discovered today because of an elevated PSA or abnormal DRE or as an incidental finding on a transurethral resection of the prostate (TURP) specimen. Patients with locally advanced disease may present with lower urinary tract symptoms, hematospermia, decreased ejaculate volume, and impotence. Patients with metastatic disease at diagnosis (25%) may present with bone pain, weight loss, anemia, shortness of breath, lymphedema, neurologic symptoms, lymphadenopathy, or urinary retention.

WORKUP

History

Inquire about bone pain, recent weight loss, shortness of breath, asymmetric swelling of lower extremities, hip or leg pain, difficulty in walking, and voiding symptoms. A family history of prostate cancer is important.

Physical Examination

A DRE by an experienced examiner and a complete physical should be performed.

Laboratory Tests

Serum PSA is the single most important test in the initial diagnosis of prostate cancer. Once a diagnosis has been made, then further workup may include a complete blood count, chemistry panel, and liver function tests including alkaline phosphatase. An enzymatic prostatic acid phosphatase is rarely helpful in the era of PSA.

Prostate Biopsy

A histologic or cytologic diagnosis must be made before undertaking any form of therapy. Two techniques are most common: core-needle biopsy and fine-needle aspiration.

■ Core-Needle Biopsy

Core-needle biopsy using a spring-loaded gun and a transrectal approach is preferred. The transrectal approach is more accurate and less painful. Complications include sepsis and bleeding. Always give prophylactic antibiotics. Ultrasound-guided transrectal biopsies have become the gold standard because of the added ability to target hypoechoic defects and randomly sample the entire gland in a systematic fashion. A transperineal approach has a lower incidence of infectious complications but makes it more difficult to obtain an accurate specimen.

■ Fine-Needle Aspiration

Fine-needle aspiration is performed using a Franzen needle and a transrectal approach. It has the lowest complication rate but does not give tissue and therefore relies on accurate cytologic interpretation and also does not provide a Gleason grade.

■ Indications for Biopsy

- A palpably suspicious DRE regardless of PSA level
- PSA greater than 4.0 ng/mL regardless of DRE or transrectal ultrasound (TRUS)
- PSA greater than the patient's age-specific range

■ Indications for Repeat Biopsy

- Persistently abnormal or rising PSA
- PSA between 4.0 and 10.0 ng/mL with a low percent free PSA (<15%)
- Evidence of high-grade prostatic intraepithelial neoplasia on a prior biopsy

Transrectal Ultrasound

TRUS aids in the localization of prostate cancers and is indispensable for accurate needle biopsy of the prostate. However, TRUS has poor sensitivity and specificity for the detection of prostate cancer. Yet many prostate cancers tend to be hypoechogenic on ultrasound and most frequently are located in the peripheral zone. Negative findings on TRUS do not negate the indications for biopsy.

■ Indications for Transrectal Ultrasound of the Prostate

- To aid prostate needle biopsy
- To measure prostate size for PSA density

Imaging Studies

Routine intravenous urography is not recommended. Pelvic imaging with computed tomography or magnetic resonance imaging is only warranted in men with a high risk of metastases (PSA >20 ng/mL, high grade and locally advanced on DRE). They are not routinely used because of low sensitivity in detecting the local extent of disease.

■ Nuclear Bone Scan

A bone scan is the most sensitive (97%) test for bony metastases. Look for multiple asymmetric areas of increased uptake in the axial skeleton. Skeletal radiographs may help confirm a positive bone scan. Positive bone scans generally precede radiographic visualization by 3 to 6 months. Serial follow-up scans, after definitive therapy, are often misleading and unnecessary. Repeat scans are indicated in the setting of a rising PSA and for new complaints of bone pain. A bone scan also provides information about possible upper tract obstruction. The probability of a positive bone scan in men with a PSA of less than 10 ng/mL is low.

■ Lymphangiograms

Lymphangiograms are rarely performed. They have only a 50% sensitivity for detecting pelvic metastasis, and proper interpretation depends on experience.

Pelvic Lymph Node Dissection

A node dissection is the most accurate means of identifying lymphatic involvement and should precede radical surgical treatment. A laparoscopic pelvic lymph node dissection is an option for the patient at high risk for metastatic disease or to stage patients before radiotherapy. Five percent to 10% of men with clinically localized prostate cancer are found to have positive pelvic lymph nodes.

TREATMENT OPTIONS

Total (Radical) Prostatectomy

Any candidates for total prostatectomy should have a better than average life expectancy by virtue of their present age (usually <70 years) and good general health. A radical retropubic prostatectomy, preceded by a negative pelvic lymph node dissection, *offers the best chance for cure* to patients with clinically localized disease. A nerve-sparing procedure can be performed to preserve potency. Complications following a radical prostatectomy are directly related to the skill and experience of the surgeon. Serious incontinence is less than 2% and impotence is less than 25%. A laparoscopic prostatectomy (hand or robotic assisted) is an option; however, insufficient data are available to demonstrate equivalent results. Laparoscopic prostatectomy is considerably more difficult and takes twice as long to perform, and regional anesthetics are contraindicated.

Radiotherapy

Irradiation has been used for curative, palliative, or prophylactic treatment for prostate cancer. Modalities include external-beam and interstitial radiation implants.

▮ External-Beam Radiotherapy

Standard external-beam radiotherapy typically delivers a total of 65 to 75 Gy to the prostate over 6 to 7 weeks. Newer techniques of three-dimensional conformal radiotherapy, including intensity-modulated radiation therapy (IMRT) and dynamic IMRT, use complex treatment planning software algorithms achieving exceedingly high doses of radiation delivered to the target, while significantly smaller doses of radiation are given to the adjacent normal tissue. Overall survival data are close to those obtained with surgery in the short term (5 years). However, long-term (10–15 years) biochemical failure rates are considerably higher than those with radical prostatectomy. Complications are generally self-limiting and mainly include diarrhea, rectal irritation, dysuria, and frequency. The appearance of impotence is often delayed and can be expected in about 50% of patients. Neoadjuvant hormonal downsizing of the prostate with luteinizing hormone–releasing hormone (LHRH) agonists decreases the target volume and is recommended for large glands.

▮ Interstitial Radiotherapy (Brachytherapy)

Interstitial radiotherapy (brachytherapy) uses the permanent implantation of radioactive seeds under ultrasound guidance. This potentially allows a more accurate and uniform seed distribution than with previous implant techniques and, thus, a more homogeneous radiation dose to the entire prostate gland. Iodine-125 (^{125}I) and palladium-103 (^{103}P) are the most common seeds used. The principal advantage of brachytherapy is its ability to theoretically deliver more radiation to the prostate with less dose to the surrounding normal tissues. Primary brachytherapy is recommended for older patients (age ≥ 70) with low PSA (<10 ng/mL), low-grade (Gleason's sum 6 or less), and low-stage (cT2a or less) prostate cancers. PSA-free survival is not as good as with radical prostatectomy and may not even be as good as with external-beam radiotherapy. Relative contraindications to brachytherapy include very large or very small prostates, severe lower urinary tract symptoms, or a prior TURP.

▮ Palliative Radiotherapy

Palliative radiotherapy (30 Gy over 10 sessions) is effective local treatment for painful skeletal metastases.

■ **Prophylactic Radiotherapy**

Prophylactic radiotherapy to weight-bearing areas such as the spine or femoral neck may help prevent pathologic fractures.

Hormonal Therapy

Normal metabolic functions of prostatic cells are androgen dependent. Testosterone is the major circulating androgen; 90% is produced by the testis (Leydig's cells) and 10% by the adrenals. Androgenic activity in the prostate results from intracytoplasmic conversion of testosterone to dihydrotestosterone (DHT) by the enzyme 5-α-reductase. Testicular testosterone production is under the control of LH from the anterior pituitary and the negative feedback effect of testosterone. The anterior pituitary is in turn under control of hypothalamic LHRH. Prostate tissue will atrophy without testicular androgen production. Adrenal androgens are insufficient to sustain normal prostatic metabolism. Prostate cancer is best viewed as a heterogeneous population of both androgen-dependent and androgen-independent cells. Suppression of testosterone stimulation results in atrophy of this androgen-dependent cell population only. The primary tumor volume will decrease by an average of 30% to 40% after androgen withdrawal. Reintroduction of androgens will result in regrowth of the tumor.

The major side effects of androgen withdrawal are loss of libido and potency. Other long-term side effects include hot flashes, osteoporosis, fatigue, loss of muscle mass, and weight gain with increased fat deposition.

Endocrine treatment of prostate cancer is purely palliative. No hormonal treatment regimen of prostate cancer has yet demonstrated improved overall survival.

■ **Methods of Androgen Suppression**

Bilateral Orchiectomy

Bilateral orchiectomy (castration) is the single most effective method of suppressing testosterone. It is safe, is immediate, and does not require continued patient compliance. Serum testosterone levels will decrease to 5% to 10% of the original levels within 3 to 12 hours after castration. Hot flashes appear to be less severe and self-limiting with castration compared with LHRH agonist therapy.

Estrogen

Estrogen administration lowers circulating testosterone levels by suppressing pituitary luteinizing hormone (LH) secretion. The most commonly used estrogen is diethylstilbestrol (DES). Doses of 5 mg/day have significant cardiovascular side effects, including deep venous thromboses. DES 1 mg orally (PO) daily (qd) is considered safe and produces castrate testosterone levels in most patients. Castrate levels of testosterone will be reached within 21 to 60 days after beginning 3 mg/day DES. Gynecomastia will develop in 70% if pretreatment radiation therapy to the breasts (8–10 Gy over 1–3 days) is not given at least 2 days before starting estrogens.

Progestins

Progestins inhibit pituitary LH release and act as an antiandrogen by binding to DHT receptors, blocking 5-α-reductase conversion of testosterone to DHT. However, low-dose DES (0.1 mg daily) must also be given to prevent suppression escape after 6 months of therapy. Megestrol acetate is the most frequently used progestin.

Luteinizing Hormone–Releasing Hormone Agonists

Leuprolide (Lupron) and goserelin (Zoladex) are superactive synthetic LHRH agonists that suppress LH and testosterone after an initial stimulation phase. The initial stimulation phase lasts 2 to 3 weeks and causes a flare phenomenon both biochemically and clinically with increased PSA and symptoms such as bone pain. The flare phenomenon can be suppressed by giving antiandrogens such as flutamide (Eulexin), bicalutamide (Casodex), or nilutamide (Nilandron) beginning at the time of initiating LHRH or 1 week before. Flare suppression is recommended for patients with a large tumor burden or symptoms of advanced disease.

LHRH agonists are injected monthly or every 3 months. Compliance can sometimes be a problem, and the cost of these medications is extremely high.

Antiandrogens

Antiandrogens block end organ action of testosterone by competing for androgen receptors. These agents include steroidal antiandrogens; cyproterone acetate and megestrol acetate; and pure antiandrogens, flutamide (Eulexin), bicalutamide (Casodex), or nilutamide (Nilandron). Pure antiandrogens are not effective as monotherapy and are used primarily to suppress the flare phenomenon of LHRH agonists or for total androgen blockade. Total androgen blockade does *not* result in a survival advantage in randomized trials.

5-α-Reductase Blockers

5-α-Reductase blockers inhibit the intracellular conversion of testosterone to DHT. These agents have not been proven useful in the treatment of prostate cancer.

Other Therapies

Other therapies include bilateral adrenalectomies, pituitary ablation (hypophysectomy), glucocorticoid suppression of ACTH, and prolactin inhibitors. None of these is recommended for patients with prostate cancer.

■ General Guidelines for Using Hormone Therapy

1. Clear benefits of early hormone therapy in terms of patient survival have not been proven. Therefore, delaying hormone therapy appears reasonable in asymptomatic patients who are still sexually active.
2. Indications for immediate treatment include pain, neurologic symptoms, bladder outlet or ureteral obstruction, anemia, weight loss, edema, or shortness of breath.
3. Hormone therapy does not prolong survival in patients with metastatic disease.
4. Total androgen blockade (i.e., blocking adrenal androgens) has *no* survival advantage.
5. Orchiectomy is the safest and most dependable method of testosterone suppression.
6. LHRH agonists should be avoided in patients with significant spinal metastases.
7. DES 1 mg PO qd is still an acceptable and cost-effective alternative for patients who refuse orchiectomy and are not at increased risk for cardiovascular side effects. Prophylactic breast irradiation is recommended. Testosterone levels should be checked if PSA fails to suppress.

Chemotherapy

Overall results from chemotherapeutic trials have been disappointing. Recent studies of docetaxel-based chemotherapy regimens in patients with androgen-independent metastatic prostate cancer have demonstrated short-term (6 to 9 months) improvement.

TREATMENT GUIDE

Local Disease

Total prostatectomy offers the best chance for a durable long-lasting cure from localized prostate cancer. Failure can only occur because of understaging the disease. All tumor within the prostate is permanently eradicated. If the prostatectomy is performed by an experienced surgeon, the side effects are generally negligible in appropriately selected patients. Patients who fail locally after a radical prostatectomy may still be eligible for cure with adjuvant external-beam radiotherapy.

External-beam radiotherapy using three-dimensional conformal techniques is an excellent primary alternative for patients with localized disease who may be older or who are poor surgical candidates. Interstitial radioactive seed implantation should be limited to patients with low-grade, low-stage disease and no contraindications. All forms of radiation therapy have the added risk of local failure in the retained prostate in addition to failure because of understaging. Total prostatectomy after local failure of radiotherapy has limited application because of the high complication rate.

Advanced or Metastatic Disease

Endocrine therapy is the primary treatment for patients with locally advanced or metastatic disease.

EMERGENCY TREATMENT

Occasionally, patients present with untreated metastatic prostate cancer and signs of incipient spinal cord compression (e.g., lower extremity weakness and lax anal sphincter tone). These patients need emergency treatment to decrease tumor mass and relieve cord compression. Motor function is lost first with spinal cord compression, and pinprick sensation is the last to go. Patients who have retained pinprick sensation may safely be given a trial of other forms of treatment before resorting to a decompression laminectomy. Neurologic consultation should be obtained.

Options

1. Emergency bilateral orchiectomies
2. Ketoconazole [400 mg PO every 8 hours (q8h)]
3. Intravenous DES (Stilphostrol)
4. Radiotherapy
5. Emergency decompression laminectomy

23 Urothelial Cancers

BLADDER CANCER

Bladder cancer is the second most common urologic malignancy, with close to 50,000 new cases and 12,000 deaths reported each year. Eighty percent of cases occur in patients older than age 50. Males are affected more commonly than females in a 3:1 ratio. Transitional cell carcinoma (TCC) accounts for 90% of these cases; squamous cell carcinoma (SCC) accounts for about 8%; and adenocarcinoma accounts for 2%. Whites are more commonly affected than blacks by a 4:1 ratio. What follows pertains to TCC, except where indicated.

Etiology

As with most cancers, no cause of bladder cancer is known. However, there is strong circumstantial evidence that environmental exposure to carcinogens plays a major role. Up to 33% of cases may be related to occupational exposures to carcinogenic aromatic amines in dye, textile, rubber, cable, printing, and plastics industries. Four proven bladder carcinogens are (a) 3-naphthylamine, (b) 4-aminobiphenyl (xenylamine), (c) 4-nitrobiphenyl, and (d) 4,4-diaminobiphenyl (benzidine). Significant nonoccupational exposures are cigarette smoking, dietary nitrosamines, *Schistosoma haematobium* infection of the bladder, and possibly caffeine, saccharin, and cyclamates. A latent period of 15 to 20 years from first exposure to carcinogens to diagnosis of a tumor is common. Familial history does not appear to be significant. It is important to take a history of risk factors so they may be removed during treatment.

Pathology

TCC is described as a field defect because the entire urothelium, from the renal pelvis to the bladder, is bathed in the urinary carcinogens. However, most tumors occur on the floor of the bladder where exposure is greatest. These tumors usually grow in a papillary fashion and are often multicentric.

Two important variants of bladder cancer are bladder papillomas and carcinoma in situ. Bladder papillomas are transitional cell tumors or Stage Ta bladder cancers with a high rate of recurrence (up to 47%). Close follow-up of these lesions is necessary because approximately 3% will progress to frank bladder cancer. Carcinoma in situ appears as a flat, nonpapillary, erythematous lesion confined to the urothelial mucosa. It is histologically characterized by severe urothelial dysplasia, is clearly more aggressive, and is associated with a poorer prognosis than papillary lesions. Carcinoma in situ has a high recurrence rate of more than 80%, most are multifocal, and progression to a higher stage and grade occurs in 50% to 75%.

Staging Nomenclature and Criteria

The pathologic stage of the cancer (i.e., depth of invasion into bladder wall) is the single most important prognostic factor. Normal histologic anatomy of the bladder includes the inner urothelium, the lamina propria, and the outer muscularis propria. Smooth muscle fibers found in the lamina propria, referred to as the muscularis mucosa, must not be confused with the true muscularis propria, which constitutes the detrusor muscle. Cancer invasion of the muscularis mucosa should not be considered true muscle invasive bladder cancer and thus should be treated differently. Uncertainty can arise in the transurethral resection specimens. The TNM classification is reviewed in the following table.

■ TNM Staging Classification—American Joint Committee on Cancer	
	Description
T	**Primary tumor**
Ta	Neoplasm confined to mucosa
Tis	Carcinoma in situ (confined to mucosa)
T1	Tumor invades submucosa/lamina propria
T2a	Tumor invades superficial muscle
T2b	Tumor invades deep muscle
T3	Tumor invades perivesical fat
T4a	Tumor invades prostate, uterus, or vagina
T4b	Tumor invades pelvic or abdominal wall
N	**Lymph nodes**
N1	Single regional lymph node, <2 cm in diameter
N2	One or more lymph nodes, none >5 cm
N3	One or more lymph nodes, >5 cm
M	**Metastases**
M1	Distant metastasis

Tumor Grade

Tumor grade refers to the histologic morphology as determined by cellular atypia, nuclear abnormalities, and the number as well as location of mitotic figures. The Mostofi three-grade system follows:

Grade 1—well-differentiated (~10% will be invasive)
Grade 2—moderately differentiated (~50% will be invasive)
Grade 3—poorly differentiated (>80% will be invasive)

Workup

▪ History

Gross hematuria is the hallmark of bladder cancer either alone or associated with irritative symptoms (frequency, urgency, and dysuria). Irritative symptoms will present alone in approximately 30% of cases, usually with invasive cancer or carcinoma in situ. Other less common presentations include flank pain (ureteral obstruction), pelvic pain (spread outside bladder), and leg edema (lymphatic involvement). A secondary urinary tract infection may be present in up to 30%.

▪ Physical Examination

The physical examination is usually unremarkable except in far advanced disease. A bimanual examination should be performed at the time of cystoscopy. A palpable tumor indicates that at least the muscular wall is involved.

▪ Laboratory Tests

Urinalysis and culture are performed to confirm hematuria and to look for evidence of infection. Even if infection is demonstrated and hematuria clears after treatment with antibiotics, further investigation should be undertaken in high-risk individuals (age, sex, industrial exposure, smoker).

▪ X-Ray Studies

An intravenous urogram should be obtained in all patients with hematuria, preferably before cystoscopy in case retrograde studies are needed to further delineate filling defects in the upper tracts. A negative cystogram phase of an intravenous urogram does not exclude a bladder tumor and therefore does not cancel the need for cystoscopy. Ureteral obstruction or bladder displacement suggests an invasive tumor. In patients with iodine contrast sensitivity, bilateral retrograde pyelograms can be performed at the time of cystoscopy. Few patients with bladder tumors will have concurrent upper tract lesions; however, one third of patients with upper tract tumors will have an associated bladder cancer.

■ Cystoscopy

Cystoscopy is the definitive study to evaluate the bladder for tumors and must be performed to evaluate hematuria properly in the adult. Carefully inspect for sessile or papillary growths. A slightly raised, red, velvetlike patch of mucosa can indicate carcinoma in situ. Attempt to view inside of diverticula if at all possible. The incidence of carcinoma in diverticula is approximately 2% to 3%.

■ Cytology

Urinary cytology may be helpful. A combined specimen of cystoscopic urine and 50 mL saline bladder washing (to preserve cellular integrity) or a voided urine specimen can be obtained. Up to 95% of patients with high-grade tumors will have positive cytologies, whereas only 50% to 75% will be positive with grade I or II neoplasms.

■ Biopsies

Tumors discovered on cystoscopy will need to be biopsied for diagnosis and treatment. Deep resection of the entire tumor with underlying muscle is necessary. Resection should be followed by superficial random cold cup biopsies from the anterior wall or dome, each lateral wall, the posterior wall, trigone, and the prostatic urethra (in males), looking for field changes consistent with carcinoma in situ. Tumors within diverticula should be removed by cold cup biopsy and fulguration or open surgery.

■ Ureteroscopy

Ureteroscopy can be used for visualization of upper tract lesions, biopsy, and fulguration of small upper tract tumors. Ureteral washings should be sent for cytology if there is suspicion of an upper tract tumor.

■ Computed Tomography Scan

Computed tomography (CT) is useful in identifying intraabdominal and pelvic lymph node enlargements of greater than 1.5 cm. A 40% false-negative rate is related to metastases insufficient to cause enlargement of lymph nodes. Skinny needle biopsy confirmation of suspected nodes is usually necessary. CT primarily serves a role in staging large or bulky bladder tumors and in serving as a baseline to assess response to radiation or chemotherapy.

■ Magnetic Resonance Imaging

Magnetic resonance imaging adds little to standard CT imaging of bladder cancer soft tissues but has become increasingly useful in determining bony involvement.

■ Flow Cytometry

Flow cytometry uses cellular material obtained from bladder washings or by mincing tissues to determine DNA ploidy of transitional cell tumors. Cell populations with hyperdiploid DNA content have been associated with the presence of malignant transitional cell tumors in 80% of cases. Flow cytometry has not been found to add much useful clinical information over conventional cytology.

Management

A general guideline to the management of transitional cell tumors of the bladder follows. Treatment options must be carefully individualized. Major prognostic factors include stage, grade, size, number of lesions, recurrence, and presence of carcinoma in situ.

■ Carcinoma in Situ (Tis)

Carcinoma in situ, despite its superficial location, has consistently demonstrated its more aggressive behavior, with 50% to 75% of cases progressing to more advanced disease, often skipping directly to dissemination. Radical cystectomy was the therapy of choice until studies demonstrated favorable response rates using intravesical bacillus Calmette-Guérin (BCG) or mitomycin C chemotherapy. Failure to respond to intravesical therapy requires consideration of radical cystectomy.

■ Superficial Bladder Cancer

Stages Ta to T1—transurethral resection is curative in most cases.
- *Stage Ta (confined to mucosa)*—recurrence occurs in 50% and progression in only 3%.
- *Stage T1 (invasion of lamina propria)*—recurrence occurs in 75% and progression in 30%. Tumor recurrence can be managed with repeat transurethral resection and prophylactic intravesical chemotherapy.

Intravesical Therapy

Instillation of immunotherapeutic or chemotherapeutic agents into the bladder with a catheter provides direct access to the tumor for therapy. The most frequent side effects of intravesical therapy are lower urinary tract symptoms for all agents.

■ Indications for Intravesical Therapy

1. Rapid tumor recurrence
2. Multicentricity
3. Progression to higher grade or invasion of the lamina propria
4. Presence of carcinoma in situ

BCG is a preparation of attenuated tubercle bacillus. Mode of action is immunologic. Response rates of up to 70% are obtained. Initial treatment is once a week intravesical instillation for 6 weeks. Maintenance therapy includes 3 weekly instillations every 6 months. BCG immunotherapy should be delayed 2 to 4 weeks after transurethral resection. Significant hematuria is a contraindication to instillation. Dose is 1 ampule TICE strain in 60 mL saline with a 2-hour dwell time. Gross hematuria and bacterial infection are contraindications to instillation.

Systemic toxicity called "BCGosis" can result from increased absorption of BCG through the bladder wall, particularly after recent transurethral resection. BCGosis is potentially dangerous and requires systemic antituberculosis therapy.

■ Management of BCG Toxicity

1. Mild local or systemic symptoms (last <24 hr)
   Local symptoms—cystitis, dysuria, gross hematuria
   Systemic symptom—malaise, fatigue, lethargy, and fever <101°F
   • Acetaminophen 650 mg PO q4h × 12–24 hr prn
   • Pyridium 200 mg PO tid
   • Anticholinergic therapy (oxybutynin 5 mg PO tid)
2. Persistent mild local or systemic symptoms (last >24 hr)
   • Isoniazid 300 mg PO qd × 3 days (day before treatment, day of treatment, and day after treatment)
   • Never give BCG when patient has gross hematuria
3. Severe life-threatening systemic toxicity (acute fever to >103°F)
   • Patient should be hospitalized
   • Blood and urine culture followed by broad-spectrum antibiotics
   • Cycloserine 250–500 mg PO bid or
   • Isoniazid 300 mg PO qd and rifampicin 600 mg PO qd

PO, orally; prn, as needed; qd, daily; q4h, every 4 hours; tid, three times a day.

α-Interferon intravesical instillation may produce responses in up to 40%. Patients may develop mild to moderate flulike symptoms. Dose is 100 million units in 50 mL normal saline weekly × 12.

Mitomycin C is obtained from *Streptomyces caespitosus*. Its mode of action is inhibition of DNA synthesis. Response rates of up to 50% are obtained. Dose is 40 mg in 60 mL water every week for 6 to 8 weeks. Maintenance is monthly × 12.

Thiotepa is an alkylating agent. Response rates of up to 50% are obtained. Dose is 30 mg in 30 mL water every week for 6 to 8 weeks. Maintenance is monthly × 12.

Leukopenia may occur. White blood cell and platelet count should be monitored.

Follow-Up for Superficial Bladder Cancer

Because of the high incidence of recurrence, all patients with superficial tumors should be closely followed with local cystoscopic surveillance every 3 months for the first year, every 6 months for the second year, and annually thereafter. Suspicious cytologies or areas of mucosa warrant bladder biopsies.

■ Muscle-Invasive Bladder Cancer—Stage T2

Surgery

Radical cystectomy and pelvic lymphadenectomy constitute the treatment of choice for both superficial and deep muscle invasive bladder cancer (Stage T2) and for patients with stage Tis/T1 disease who have failed two courses of intravesical therapy or for persistent high grade 3 lesions. Partial cystectomy has been successful for T2a lesions localized to the dome of the bladder, with 5-year survival rates of 50% to 70%.

Radiation

High-energy, external-beam irradiation has been unsuccessful as the sole mode of therapy for bladder cancer. However, some data suggest an advantage to combination preoperative irradiation followed by cystectomy. Radiation therapy is primarily reserved for patients who refuse cystectomy.

Chemotherapy

Half of all patients, independent of treatment with surgery and/or radiation, fail therapy. The primary cause of treatment failure in bladder cancer is widespread disseminated disease. Adjuvant combination chemotherapy with methotrexate, vinblastine, Adriamycin, and cisplatin (M-VAC) can be undertaken for patients with stage T3/T4 or node-positive disease. Renal dysfunction is often the dose-limiting factor; therefore, preservation of an obstructed kidney may be important if M-VAC chemotherapy is contemplated.

Newer agents such as gemcitabine, paclitaxel, and docetaxel have shown variable degrees of effectiveness. Metastatic disease has a poor prognosis, with more than 50% dead within 1 year.

SQUAMOUS CELL CARCINOMA

SCC accounts for less than 8% of all primary bladder cancers. Most patients have advanced invasive disease at presentation, and their prognosis is poor. Risk factors for the development of SCC include chronic urinary tract infections, urinary calculi, stricture disease, inflammation, chronic indwelling Foley catheters, diverticula, and schistosomiasis. The urothelium responds to chronic irritation, inflammation, or infection with squamous metaplasia; however, there is no clear evidence linking this with the development of SCC.

Diagnosis

Diagnosis and clinical staging of SCC are identical to those of TCC. The tumors are graded pathologically on a scale of 1 to 4. Stage-for-stage survival rates are comparable with those for TCC; however, most patients present with advanced disease.

Treatment

The infrequent, well-differentiated, superficial tumor can be managed by transurethral resection. Locally invasive tumors are managed by radical cystectomy. A urethrectomy is usually not indicated because carcinoma in situ is uncommon with SCC. Patients with lymph node involvement generally survive only 3 to 6 months. No effective chemotherapy has yet been identified.

ADENOCARCINOMA

Adenocarcinoma of the bladder is an extremely uncommon tumor, responsible for less than 2% of all bladder tumors. It tends to be locally aggressive and is diagnosed at an advanced stage (85%) with a uniformly poor prognosis. The appearance of primary vesical adenocarcinoma has been associated with metaplastic changes induced by irritation, infection, and obstruction, which often produce a premalignant state of cystitis glandularis. These tumors may also arise from a urachal origin or be metastatic from the gastrointestinal or female genital tract. Seventy percent of patients present with hematuria, and most patients will give a history of chronic urinary tract infections. Patients with exstrophy of the bladder have had a high association of development of adenocarcinoma of the bladder.

UPPER TRACT TRANSITIONAL CELL TUMORS

Only about 4% of all TCCs are located in the renal pelvis or ureter. The other 96% are located in the bladder (90%) and urethra (6%). Additionally, approximately one third of patients with an upper tract TCC will develop an associated lower tract tumor, and about 2% to 4% will develop a tumor in the contralateral collecting system.

Patients most commonly present with gross hematuria, which occurs in 70% to 80%. Flank pain is the second most common complaint. The average age at diagnosis is 60 to 65 years; half of the patients will have only superficial disease and the other half more advanced disease. The natural history of this disease has shown a high correlation between the tumor stage and grade and the prognosis. Risk factors include chemical carcinogens and cigarette smoking. Abuse of analgesic containing phenacetin or aspirin is associated with a nine times increased risk of TCC of the renal pelvis.

Diagnosis

Diagnosis is generally made using a combination of modalities including excretory urography, retrograde ureteropyelography, cytology, brush biopsies, and ureteropyeloscopic visualization and biopsy as needed. Persistence and reevaluation of patients with recurrent unexplained gross hematuria should be emphasized. Staging studies include CT and/or magnetic resonance imaging.

	TNM Staging Classification—American Joint Committee on Cancer
	Description
T	**Primary tumor**
Ta	Neoplasm confined to mucosa
Tis	Carcinoma in situ (confined to mucosa)
T1	Tumor invades submucosa/lamina propria
T2	Tumor invades muscle
T3	Tumor invades periureteral/peripelvic fat or renal parenchyma
T4	Tumor invades adjacent organs
N	**Lymph nodes**
N1	Single regional lymph node, <2 cm in diameter
N2	One or more lymph nodes, none <5 cm
N3	One or more lymph nodes, >5 cm
M	**Metastases**
M1	Distant metastasis

Tumor Grade

Grade 1—well-differentiated
Grade 2—moderately differentiated
Grade 3–4—poorly differentiated—undifferentiated

Management of Upper Tract Transitional Cell Tumors

Complete nephroureterectomy with excision of a cuff of bladder remains the standard treatment for stage Ta to T4 because of the high incidence of recurrence with more conservative management. Exceptions to this are as follows:

1. Low grade–low stage distal ureteral tumors can be safely managed with a more conservative distal ureterectomy, excision of a bladder cuff, and reimplant.
2. Patients with multiple bilateral tumors or a solitary kidney would also warrant attempts at more conservative open renal parenchyma-sparing operations or endoscopic management with laser ablation.

Chemotherapy

Chemotherapy using M-VAC appears to be effective adjuvant therapy for patients with nodal disease.

■ Follow-Up

Follow-up should be performed every 3 months for the first year and every 6 months thereafter; it should include a chest radiograph, complete blood count, chemistry panel, urinalysis, and urine cytology. An intravenous urogram and cystoscopy should be performed each year. CT or magnetic resonance imaging would be helpful in evaluating the retroperitoneum.

Kidney Tumors

BENIGN SOLID TUMORS

Renal Cortical Adenomas

Renal cortical adenomas are benign tumors of the renal cortex that are generally discovered incidentally. They have been distinguished from renal cell carcinomas (RCCs) in the past primarily by their small size: less than 3 cm in diameter. The designation of these tumors as benign adenomas has been questioned because they are histologically indistinguishable from RCCs. It has been reasoned that all tubular cell adenomas are malignant and simply represent an early stage of renal carcinoma growth. These tumors should be treated as small RCCs.

Renal Oncocytoma

Renal oncocytoma is generally a benign, unifocal renal tumor that averages 5 to 8 cm in diameter; however, the presence of malignant elements has been known to occur. Its presentation is usually asymptomatic, with the majority being discovered incidentally. It can have a somewhat typical "spoke-wheel" appearance on angiogram, but this is uncertain. Partial or radical nephrectomy is the safest method of treatment because of the unreliability of differentiating it from RCC preoperatively.

Angiomyolipomas (Renal Hamartoma)

Angiomyolipomas are generally benign tumors, are frequently bilateral or multiple, and are often associated with tuberous sclerosis. Histologically, they are composed of fat cells, blood vessels, and sheets of smooth muscle cells. Profuse internal hemorrhage can occur. Its angiographic pattern is not characteristic; however, it has a distinctive fat content on computed tomography (CT) that is usually diagnostic. Asymptomatic lesions smaller than 4 cm should be followed with yearly ultrasound examinations. Larger tumors should be considered for embolization or renal-sparing surgery. Conservative surgical therapy is necessary because of frequent bilaterality and multiplicity.

Other Rare Benign Renal Tumors

Fibroma, lipoma, leiomyoma, angioma, rhabdomyoma, neurofibroma, dermoid tumors, and tumors of endometriosis are other rare benign renal tumors.

Pseudotumors

Pseudotumors are normal variants of functioning renal tissue that can occasionally appear as a questionable renal mass on intravenous urography (IVU) or ultrasound. They include fetal lobulations, column of Bertin, dromedary hump, hilar lip or uncus, and nodular compensatory hypertrophy. A CT scan will generally differentiate a true tumor from a pseudotumor. However, if one suspects an equivocal renal mass to be a pseudotumor, then a dimercaptosuccinic acid (DMSA) renal scan may be helpful. A pseudotumor will appear as normal homogeneous functioning kidney, whereas a true renal mass will appear as a focal defect within the renal parenchyma (sensitivity 95%).

MALIGNANT TUMORS

Renal Cell Carcinoma (Hypernephroma, Renal Adenocarcinoma)

RCC is the most common solid renal tumor (90%). It is primarily a tumor of adults (age 40–60 years), with a 2:1 male predominance. Approximately 30,000 new diagnoses are made each year in the United States, and 12,000 deaths from it are recorded. It arises from cells of the proximal convoluted tubule with no known cause. These are typically round tumors of varying size with a pseudocapsule and areas of hemorrhage and necrosis, and they often displace or invade the collecting system. Local extension occasionally occurs despite Gerota's fascia. Tumor thrombus into the renal vein is frequent and may extend into the vena cava. Metastatic spread is to lung, liver, bone, brain, and subcutaneous tissues.

■ **Presentation**

Because of its retroperitoneal location, symptoms such as the classic triad of pain, hematuria, and flank mass occur only rarely today and generally indicate advanced disease. More than 50% of these tumors are presenting as asymptomatic incidental findings on IVU, abdominal ultrasound, or CT scans. Nevertheless, the more frequent findings are pain (41%), hematuria (36%), weight loss (36%), flank mass (24%), hypertension (20%), hypercalcemia (13%), and erythrocytosis (3%). Some paraneoplastic syndromes may occur as a result of renal tumor production of 1,25 dihydroxycholecalciferol, rennin, erythropoietin, and other hormone substances. Hepatic dysfunction without evidence of hepatic metastasis (Stauffer's syndrome) can occur in up to 20% of patients. Epidemiologic studies suggest tobacco smoking as a likely cause.

Patients with Von Hippel–Lindau disease frequently get RCC in addition to pheochromocytomas, retinal angiomas, and hemangioblastomas of the brain and spinal cord.

■ **Diagnosis**

The renal tumor must first be differentiated from the more common benign renal cysts. Ultrasound and CT scan can effectively define the solid or cystic nature of the mass. Complete evaluation of the cystic renal mass is described in Chapter 15. Fine-needle aspiration or biopsy of a solid renal mass has little value except when lymphoma or metastases to the kidney is suspected from another primary. These biopsies have a high false-negative rate.

Intravenous Urography

IVU should be performed to fully evaluate the upper and lower urinary tract.

Abdominal Computed Tomography

A CT scan without and with intravenous (IV) contrast (renal protocol) is the method of choice to evaluate a renal mass. Any mass that enhances with IV contrast should be considered an RCC until proven otherwise. CT also provides accurate information on renal vein and inferior vena cava involvement, lymph node metastases, and perirenal extension to adjacent organs.

Magnetic Resonance Imaging

Magnetic resonance imaging (MRI) can help differentiate solid and cystic renal masses and is particularly useful in patients who cannot receive IV contrast agents. Enhancement following IV gadolinium diethylenetriamine pentaacetic acid (GDPA) on T1 images of an MRI indicates vascularity and helps identify RCC.

MRI has become the best study to evaluate the IVC for tumor thrombus.

Selective Renal Arteriography

Selective renal arteriography was the standard diagnostic test for RCC because of its classic angiographic picture of neovascularity, venous pooling, arteriovenous fistulae, and capsular vessels. Even hypovascular renal cell tumors could be differentiated by infusion of epinephrine that will constrict normal but not tumor vessels. However, arteriography is primarily reserved for patients with solitary kidneys to gain knowledge of the vascular anatomy for planning conservative surgical excision.

■ Metastatic Workup

Metastatic workup should include routine chest radiograph, IVU, CT, liver function tests, and serum calcium. A bone scan should be obtained in any patient with skeletal pain or other evidence of metastatic disease.

■ Staging Systems

Staging systems used in the United States include the simpler, but less accurate, Robson's classification, and the more complicated, but precise, TNM system. Both are included here.

■ Robson's Classification

Stage I—tumor within renal capsule
Stage II—outside capsule but within Gerota's fascia
Stage III—involvement of regional lymph nodes, renal vein, or vena cava
Stage IV—adjacent organs or distant metastases

■ TNM Staging Classification—American Joint Committee on Cancer

	Description	Robson's Stage
T	Primary tumor	
T1	Tumor ≤7 cm limited to kidney	I
T2	Tumor >7 cm limited to kidney	I
T3	Tumor extends into major veins, adrenal, or perirenal fat	
T3a	Tumor invades adrenal or perirenal fat but within Gerota's fascia	II
T3b	Tumor grossly into renal vein or vena cava	III
T3c	Tumor into vena cava above diaphragm	III
T4	Tumor invades beyond Gerota's fascia	IV
N	Lymph nodes	

■ **Treatment**

Surgery

Surgery is the most effective treatment for primary RCC. Traditionally, radical nephrectomy with early ligation of the renal artery and vein and removal of the entire kidney including Gerota's fascia and the accompanying adrenal gland has been standard treatment. However, the increasing number of incidental small renal tumors diagnosed by ultrasound and CT scans has led to greater use of nephron-sparing surgery. Partial nephrectomy had generally been reserved for tumors in solitary kidneys. Nephron-sparing surgery is now acceptable with single, small, peripheral tumors less than 4 cm and a normal contralateral kidney.

In addition to standard surgical approaches, increasing use of laparoscopy and cryoablation is now common.

T1 to T3a—radical nephrectomy (excision of the kidney and adrenal including Gerota's fascia) with a limited regional lymphadenectomy and early ligation of the artery and vein is standard therapy. Nephron-sparing surgery is used with appropriate indications (small peripheral T1a tumors).

T3b to T4—patients with only renal vein or inferior vena cava thrombus appear to benefit from radical nephrectomy. Regional lymph node or adjacent organ involvement is a dire prognostic sign. However, because radical nephrectomy is the most effective therapy for renal cell cancer, extended radical surgery may be appropriate if complete excision is contemplated.

Metastatic disease—distant metastatic disease is present in 30% of patients at the time of diagnosis. These patients have an average survival of only 4 months, and only 10% survive 1 year. The use of the term "adjunctive nephrectomy" in this group was adopted in the past because of the rare cases of spontaneous regression of metastases that had occurred after nephrectomy. However, regression can be expected in less than 1% of patients, which advises against such therapy. "Palliative nephrectomy" is reserved for patients with severe hemorrhage, pain, or paraneoplastic syndromes.

Radiation Therapy

Preoperative or postoperative irradiation has not been shown to influence overall survival.

Chemotherapy

RCC remains resistant to currently available chemotherapeutic agents.

Hormonal Therapy

No report has proved the efficacy of progesterone therapy in the treatment of RCC.

Immunotherapy

Both active and passive immunotherapy has shown promise in the treatment of advanced RCC. Immunotherapeutic protocols using interferon-α or interleukin (IL)-2 in patients with nonbulky metastatic disease after nephrectomy have had favorable responses.

Observation

Observation of small renal tumors less than 3 cm in the elderly or poor surgical risk patient with serial renal imaging at 6-month or 1-year intervals is reasonable management in this setting.

Renal Sarcomas

Renal sarcomas account for only 2% of malignant renal tumors, and 60% of these are leiomyosarcomas. Differentiation from RCC is difficult or impossible until surgery. Radical nephrectomy is the treatment. Prognosis is poor without adjuvant chemotherapy.

Hemangiopericytomas

Hemangiopericytomas are highly vascular tumors that often secrete renin and may grow to a large size. Some 15% are malignant. Radical nephrectomy is the appropriate treatment.

Metastatic Renal Tumors

Usually cancers metastatic to the kidney are discovered at autopsy except for lymphoblastomas. Because they are a metastasis, removal is not indicated.

Lymphoblastomas

Lymphoid malignancies of the kidney are generally a manifestation of the systemic disease and should be treated as such. Nephrectomy is not indicated.

WILMS' TUMOR

Nephroblastoma or Wilms' tumor accounts for 95% of all urinary tract malignancies occurring in childhood, followed by RCC representing only 3%. Approximately 450 new cases occur in the United States each year. Ninety percent of these occur in children younger than 7 years, with a median age at diagnosis of 3 years. Nephroblastoma, also referred to as renal embryoma, is believed to arise from abnormal proliferation of remnants of immature kidney (metanephric blastema) within the kidney. It appears to have little familial tendency (1%–2%); however, it has been associated with other anomalies, including aniridia (1%), hemihypertrophy (3%), and genitourinary defects (4%).

Pathology

Wilms' tumor is characteristically a solitary, unilateral mass with a fleshy tan cut surface and variable areas of hemorrhage and necrosis. Venous invasion occurs in up to 20% of cases. Histologically it is composed of primitive tubules and glomerular structures in a background of stromal components and undifferentiated blastemal tissue. Three unfavorable histologic types comprise about 10% of all cases: (a) anaplasia, (b) rhabdoid tumor, and (c) clear cell sarcoma (also known as bone-metastasizing Wilms' tumor).

Major indicators of poor prognosis include unfavorable histology, distant metastases (lung, liver, bone, brain), and lymph node involvement at time of diagnosis. Other less clear prognostic factors include age (>2 years), tumor weight (>250 g), extrarenal vessel extension, direct abdominal extension, and operative spillage.

Presentation

Children appearing otherwise well will present with an enlarging, smooth abdominal mass confined to one side of the abdomen with hypertension (60%) or microscopic hematuria (25%). The differential diagnosis for an abdominal mass in a child includes hydronephrosis, multicystic kidney diseases, neuroblastoma, Wilms' tumor, splenomegaly, lymphoma, and mesenteric cysts (see Chapter 15).

Diagnosis

The diagnosis of Wilms' tumor is made radiologically by ultrasound and confirmed by CT scan or MRI. It must be differentiated from hydronephrosis, polycystic kidney, and neuroblastoma.

Treatment

Because of effective, modern multimodal therapies including surgery, radiation, and chemotherapy, survivals approaching 100% can be expected with Wilms' tumor. Protocols for managing Wilms' tumor have been extensively studied by the National Wilms' Tumor Study (NWTS) group. The latest recommendations of the NWTS (presently NWTS-5) should be reviewed.

■ Surgery

A nephrectomy is initial therapy for most children with Wilms' tumor. The contralateral kidney must be inspected for bilaterality before proceeding with nephrectomy. Large tumors should be shrunk with chemotherapy and/or radiotherapy preoperatively. A regional lymph node sampling should be performed for staging purposes.

■ Radiotherapy

Preoperative radiotherapy decreases the incidence of intraoperative tumor rupture but does not affect survival. Postoperative radiotherapy to the flank is routinely given to all children with unfavorable histology.

■ Chemotherapy

Chemotherapeutic regimens include dactinomycin, vincristine, doxorubicin, and cyclophosphamide and should begin almost immediately postoperatively.

Chapter 25

Adrenals

ANATOMY

The adrenal glands are two small, triangular, retroperitoneal structures, weighing 3 to 5 grams, with a fascial covering provided by a superior extension of Gerota's fascia. The right adrenal blood supply comes mainly from the inferior adrenal artery off the right renal artery, the middle adrenal artery off the aorta, and the superior adrenal artery off the inferior phrenic artery. The left adrenal blood supply comes mainly from the middle adrenal artery arising from the aorta and smaller superior and inferior adrenal arteries. The very short right adrenal vein empties directly into the vena cava, whereas the left adrenal vein empties into the left renal vein, lateral to the aorta and medial to the gonadal artery. Lymphatic drainage of both glands is primarily to the lateral aortic lymph nodes just above the level of the renal arteries and anterior to the crura of the diaphragm.

PHYSIOLOGY

The outer cortical zona glomerulosa produces aldosterone under the influence of angiotensin II and the renin–angiotensin system (see Renin–angiotensin–aldosterone System in Chapter 31). Aldosterone acts at the distal tubule to cause sodium retention and potassium secretion. Hyperkalemia is an important independent stimulus to aldosterone secretion.

The middle zona fasciculata and inner zona reticularis secrete primarily cortisol and dehydroepiandrosterone (DHEA) under the influence of pituitary adrenocorticotropic hormone (ACTH). Pituitary ACTH is under continuous feedback inhibition by cortisol. 17-Ketogenic steroids (17-KGSs) are metabolites of cortisol, whereas 17-ketosteroids (17-KSs) are metabolites of adrenal androgens (DHEA).

The adrenal medulla chromaffin cells function as a giant presynaptic sympathetic nerve ending secreting catecholamines, norep-

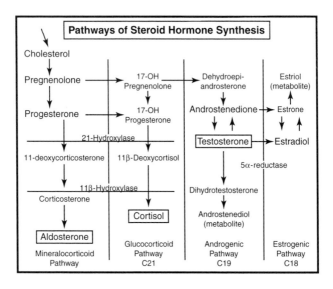

Pathways of Steroid Hormone Synthesis

inephrine (20%), and epinephrine (80%). Vanillylmandelic acid (VMA) is a major catecholamine degradation product formed by the combined action of catechol-O-methyl transferase and monoamine oxidase.

PATHOLOGY

Cushing's Syndrome

Cushing's syndrome is a clinical entity characterized by plethoric facies, bruising, truncal obesity, change in appearance, purplish cutaneous striae, hypertension, osteoporosis, hypokalemia, and poor wound healing as a result of hypersecretion of cortisol. A 24-hour urine sample demonstrating hyperexcretion of cortisol is the most reliable test.

■ Etiology

Cushing's Disease (75%)

Hypersecretion of ACTH by a pituitary adenoma unresponsive to cortisol negative feedback produces adrenal hyperplasia. Cortisol levels will be suppressed by a low-dose dexamethasone test (0.5 mg q6h for 2 days). Treatment is transsphenoidal hypophysectomy or bilateral adrenalectomy.

Ectopic ACTH (<5%)

Extra-adrenal ACTH-producing tumors are unresponsive to cortisol negative feedback and arise from malignant carcinomas in lung, breast, ovary, gastrointestinal tract, and kidney. Most common are oat cell bronchogenic carcinomas, thymic tumors, or islet cell tumors of the pancreas. Treatment is surgical excision of the tumor.

Adrenal Adenoma (20%)

This condition presents with autonomous hypersecretion of cortisol and low serum ACTH levels. These are occasionally adenocarcinomas that are radioresistant and unresponsive to chemotherapy. Adrenal adenomas are generally from 2 to 5 cm, whereas adrenal carcinomas are usually larger than 6 cm. Treatment is radical adrenalectomy and lymphadenectomy.

Aldosteronoma (Conn's Syndrome)

Aldosterone hypersecretion owing to an adrenal adenoma or hyperplasia is characterized by hypertension, hypokalemic alkalosis, and low plasma renin activity (PRA). Aldosteronomas are small tumors, usually less than 3 cm, occurring between ages 30 and 60 years, and are more common in female than in male patients (2:1). Primary hyperaldosteronism accounts for fewer than 1% of all cases of hypertension.

■ Major Criteria for Diagnosis

1. Hypertension
2. Hypokalemia in absence of diuretics
3. High aldosterone output with high sodium intake
4. Suppressed plasma renin levels that fail to increase under conditions of upright position and restricted sodium intake

■ Localization

Localization of adenomas is made with computed tomography (CT) and magnetic resonance imaging (MRI).

■ Treatment

Surgical removal is indicated if a discrete tumor is identified or if medical management fails. If the tumor has not been identified preoperatively, explore the left adrenal first (tumors are found three times more often in the left adrenal). If no tumor is found, explore the right adrenal; if still no tumor is found, then a left adrenalectomy is appropriate with perhaps a partial or total right followed by cortisol-replacement therapy. Correct potassium deficits before surgery.

Adrenal Cysts

Adrenal cysts are rare, usually incidental, findings but may become large and symptomatic.

■ Classification

1. Pseudocyst (39%) formed from liquefaction of old blood clots secondary to hemorrhage
2. Endothelial cysts (45%) lined by smooth endothelium filled with lymphogenous fluid
3. Epithelial cysts (9%)
4. Parasitic cysts (7%) secondary to echinococcal disease

■ Diagnosis

Diagnosis is made with abdominal CT, MRI, and ultrasound [eggshell calcifications (15%) need not imply malignancy].

■ Treatment

Treatment is surgical excision if symptomatic.

Adrenal Carcinomas

Adrenal carcinomas are rare tumors occurring at any age and are usually larger than 6 cm when first discovered. Eighty percent are functioning tumors, and the most common clinical manifestations are Cushing's syndrome or virilization or both, usually in female patients. An aldosterone-producing carcinoma is occasionally found. Patients with adrenal cancer commonly excrete large amounts of adrenal androgens regardless of whether the tumor causes Cushing's syndrome or virilization. These are highly malignant neoplasms that metastasize to the lungs, liver, and lymph nodes. The 3-year survival rate is less than 25%.

■ Diagnosis

Diagnosis is made by finding high levels of plasma DHEA and urinary 17-KS or high urinary free cortisol levels.

■ Localization

Localization is determined by using abdominal CT and T_2-weighted MRI.

■ **Treatment**

Treatment is surgical excision if the tumor is functioning or larger than 6 cm. Glucocorticoid replacement is necessary in functioning adrenal carcinomas because the contralateral adrenal is usually suppressed. Radiotherapy and chemotherapy are largely useless. A 34% response rate can be seen with mitotane (ortho-*para*-DDD), but no survival increase has been observed.

TUMORS ARISING FROM NEURAL CREST CELLS

Pheochromocytomas

Pheochromocytomas are rare, usually benign, tumors arising from chromaffin cells in the adrenal medulla, most commonly with a varied clinical presentation owing to hypersecretion of norepinephrine and epinephrine.

Pheochromocytomas are said to follow the "rule of 10s"—10% are malignant, 10% are multiple, 10% are bilateral, and 10% are extra-adrenal. The 10% extra-adrenal are most often found near the renal pedicles, occasionally in the organ of Zuckerkandl at the aortic bifurcation, and rarely in the thorax or wall of the bladder.

■ **Presentation**

Pheochromocytomas present in adults in the fifth and sixth decades with sustained (two thirds) and/or paroxysmal hypertension (sudden anxiety, diaphoresis, palpitation, and headaches accompanying sudden increases in blood pressure). Five percent are associated with familial syndromes such as (a) multiple endocrine adenomatosis (MEA) type II, with medullary carcinoma of the thyroid, (b) neurofibromatosis, and (c) von Hippel–Lindau syndrome.

■ **Diagnosis**

Measure 24-hour urinary free catecholamines and catecholamine metabolites: VMA, normetanephrine, and metanephrine. Check plasma norepinephrine, epinephrine, and dopamine.

■ **Localization**

Most are larger than 2 cm and can be readily demonstrated with abdominal CT. The characteristically bright T_2-weighted image on MRI scans can be effective in identifying pheochromocytomas. Selective venous sampling for catecholamines and arteriography is sometimes necessary. *Meta*-iodobenzylguanidine (MIBG) scan is useful in search of residual or multiple pheochromocytomas.

Note: Patients must be pretreated with α-blockers before radiographic contrast studies, which have been known to cause release of catecholamines.

■ Treatment

Treatment is surgical excision. Volume expand the patient before surgery, and reduce the blood pressure with titration of an α-blocker, such as oral phenoxybenzamine (20–40 mg/day initially). Complete excision of metastatic foci is recommended. The overall survival for malignant pheochromocytomas is 35% at 5 years.

Ganglioneuromas

Ganglioneuromas are benign tumors arising from mature neural crest cells of sympathetic ganglia or adrenal medulla in children. A distinct syndrome of weight loss, abdominal distention, hypertension, and chronic diarrhea is often found. Urinary free catecholamines and VMA may be elevated. Treatment is surgical excision.

Neuroblastomas

Neuroblastomas are malignant tumors that arise from immature neural crest tissue in the adrenal medulla or sympathetic ganglia. They are the most common solid tumor in children.
- 70% are first seen with metastases—poor prognosis.
- 50% to 70% arise in the adrenal medulla.
- 50% are diagnosed during the first 2 years of life.

■ Clinical Presentation

Clinical presentation includes an abdominal mass, abdominal pain, weight loss, anemia, fever, and gastrointestinal disturbances. Metastases are to bone, liver, lungs, and brain (≤70% of bone marrow aspirates are positive), and the tumors are often calcified. Urinary catecholamine levels including dopamine, VMA, and homovanillic acid (HVA) are usually elevated.

■ Treatment

Treatment is complete surgical excision when possible, with use of preoperative and/or postoperative radiotherapy when needed.

WORKUP OF ADRENAL MASSES

How to deal with the increasing number of incidental adrenal masses found on CT, MRI, or ultrasound is problematic and controversial. All patients with solid adrenal masses should probably undergo some level of biochemical assessment (electrolytes and a 24-hour urine sample measuring cortisol, VMA, and 17-ketosteroids). Tumors larger than 5 cm should be removed. Functioning tumors 5 cm or smaller should be considered for surgical removal. Nonfunctioning tumors 5 cm or smaller should be monitored.

Differential Diagnosis

- Metastatic carcinoma
- Adrenal cysts
- Functioning adrenal adenoma or carcinoma (tumors secreting cortisol or aldosterone and pheochromocytomas)
- Nonfunctioning adrenal adenoma or carcinoma (myelolipomas and malignant adrenal cortical tumors)

History

Look for symptoms of a functioning tumor (e.g., cushingoid appearance, hypertension, or virilization).

Diagnostic Imaging

- Abdominal CT with intravenous (IV) contrast
- MRI with T_2-weighted images
- Ultrasound if cyst is suspected
- Needle aspiration of equivocal cyst

24-Hour Urine Measurements

- 17-KGS: cortisol metabolites
- 17-KS: metabolites of adrenal androgens (increased levels suggest adrenal carcinoma)
- Total free (unconjugated) catecholamines
- Increased VMA in pheochromocytomas, ganglioneuromas, and neuroblastomas
- Urinary cortisol levels

Serum Measurements

- Free cortisol and ACTH
- Aldosterone and PRA
- Potassium, sodium, CO_2

Special Tests

- Dexamethasone suppression test (to rule out Cushing's disease)
- Adrenal venography (aids in localizing aldosteronomas)

MANAGEMENT OF ADRENAL MASS

Indications for Surgical Removal

- Functioning adrenal mass
- Mass larger than 5 cm on CT scan
- Mass 3 to 5 cm on CT with high T_2-weighted image on MRI
- Growing adrenal cyst

Indications for Watchful Follow-up

- Mass 5 cm or smaller on CT with low T_2-weighted image on MRI
- Stable adrenal cyst

PATHOLOGY

Testicular cancers are rare overall, yet they are the most common solid tumor of young adult males. Approximately 8,000 new cases occur annually, with 390 deaths in the United States. Primarily because of effective chemotherapy, they have become the most curable of all cancers. Germ cell cancers account for 90% to 95% of all primary testicular neoplasms. No clear etiologic or genetic factors have been defined; however, 10% of patients have a history of an undescended testis, 50% of which were intraabdominal. Testis cancers will be bilateral in 2% to 3% of cases, either concurrent or in succession. Except for seminoma, generally a rapid growth rate is found, with doubling times of 10 to 30 days. Testis tumors are broadly classified as either seminomas or nonseminomas (choriocarcinoma, embryonal, or teratocarcinoma).

■ Peak Age Incidence (Age 20–40 YR)	
Yolk Sac Tumors	**Infants and Children**
Choriocarcinoma	Age 20–30 yr
Embryonal or teratocarcinoma	Age 25–30 yr
Seminoma	Age 30–40 yr
Malignant lymphomas	Age >50 yr

TUMOR MARKERS

Many germ cell tumors produce specific oncofetal protein markers, either α-fetoprotein (AFP) or human chorionic gonadotropin (hCG), which can be detected in the patient's serum or tissues. Ninety percent of patients with nonseminomatous testis tumors will have elevations of one or both markers, and 5% to 10% of pure seminomas will demonstrate elevations of hCG only. The amount of tumor burden is proportional to the degree of marker elevation.

Human Chorionic Gonadotropin

hCG is a 38,000 MW double-chain glycoprotein with α- and β-components, normally secreted by the syncytiotrophoblastic cells of the placenta. hCG is elevated in all patients with choriocarcinoma, in 40% to 60% of embryonal carcinomas, and in 5% to 10% of pure seminomas. Its α-subunit is similar to those of luteinizing hormone, follicle-stimulating hormone, and thyroid-stimulating hormone; therefore, antibodies to the β-subunit must be used for measurement. It has a metabolic half-life of 24 hours, and normal adult levels should be less than 5 mIU/mL.

α-Fetoprotein

AFP is a 70,000 MW single-chain glycoprotein normally secreted by the fetal yolk sac. It is also produced by trophoblastic cells of embryonal carcinoma and yolk sac tumors. It is *not* made by pure choriocarcinoma or seminoma. Elevated AFP is found in 50% to 70% of nonseminomatous testis tumors. It has a half-life of 4 to 6 days, and normal adult levels should be less than 40 ng/mL.

Lactate Dehydrogenase

Lactate dehydrogenase (LDH) is a nonspecific cellular enzyme that can be used in monitoring patients with metastatic germ cell tumors.

METASTASES

More than half of patients with testicular tumors present with metastatic disease.

Local Metastases

Local metastatic spread is generally predictable and progresses in a systematic pattern to the regional lymphatics at the level of the renal hilum. Left-sided drainage is primarily to the paraaortic and preaortic areas at the level of L2 (left-to-right crossover has not been reported). Right-sided drainage is primarily to the interaortocaval, precaval, and preaortic areas at the level of L2 (right-to-left crossover is common). Retrograde spread to ipsilateral common and external iliac nodes can occur with advanced disease.

Distant Metastases

Distant metastatic spread is most commonly hematogenous to the lungs, liver, brain, bones, and kidney.

STAGING SYSTEM

Clinical staging of testis cancer is essential for the appropriate decisions for treatment. The American Joint Committee on Cancer tumor-node-metastasis system is noted below.

American Joint Committee on Cancer Tumor-Node-Metastasis Staging for Testicular Cancer	
Stage	**Description**
Tis	Intratubular tumor (carcinoma in situ)
T1	Tumor limited to testis
T2	Tumor extends outside tunic albuginea or shows vascular–lymphatic invasion
T3	Tumor invades spermatic cord
T4	Tumor invades scrotum
N1	Regional lymph nodes <2 cm and/or ≤5 nodes
N2	Regional lymph nodes of ≤5 cm or >5 nodes involved
N3	Lymph nodes >5 cm
M1a	Nonregional lymph nodes or pulmonary metastases
M1b	Other distant metastases

CLASSIFICATION OF HISTOLOGIC TYPES

Sixty percent of germ cell tumors are of a single cell type, whereas 40% will be mixed. Germ cell tumor types tend to parallel their normal developmental counterparts, as illustrated.

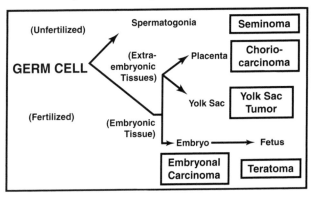

Single Cell Type (60%)

■ Seminomas (35%)

Seminomas tend to grow in sheets of cells at a slower rate than other germ cell tumors. At presentation, 75% will be confined to the testis, 15% will involve regional lymphatics, and 10% will have already spread to distant lymph nodes or viscera. Overall survival is 85%, with more than 90% survival when the tumor is confined to the testis. The tumor is very radiosensitive. hCG is produced by 5% to 10%, but *no* pure seminoma produces AFP. An elevated AFP level excludes the diagnosis of pure seminoma.

Three Subtypes

1. Classic seminoma (85%)
2. Anaplastic seminoma (10%)—generally considered a more aggressive tumor with greater metastatic potential
3. Spermatocytic seminoma (5%)—variable metastatic potential

■ Embryonal Carcinoma (20%)

Embryonal carcinoma is a grayish white fleshy tumor, often with extensive hemorrhage and necrosis. It produces both hCG and AFP.

■ Teratomas (5%)

Teratomas contain derivatives of all three cell layers: ectoderm (squamous epithelium or neuronal tissue), endoderm (gastrointestinal or respiratory tissue), and mesoderm (bone, cartilage, or muscle). They appear as clear or mucinous cystic areas interspersed with solid tissue, including bone, muscle, or cartilage. Immature and more mature varieties are differentiated. They have a somewhat less malignant potential. Pure teratomas do not produce hCG or AFP.

■ Choriocarcinomas (<1%)

Choriocarcinomas are highly malignant and appear as small grayish white tumors with central areas of hemorrhage. Both syncytiotrophoblasts and cytotrophoblasts must be demonstrated histologically to make the diagnosis. High titers of hCG are always present. Pure forms do not produce AFP. They often metastasize early.

■ Yolk Sac Tumor (<1%)

Also known as endodermal sinus tumor or orchioblastoma, this tumor occurs in a pure form primarily in children, whereas in adults, it can frequently occur in combination with other histologic types. It is the most common testicular neoplasm in infants and children. AFP is produced in high titers.

Mixed-Cell Types (40%)

■ Teratocarcinoma (20%)

Teratocarcinoma is a combination of teratoma and embryonal carcinoma. It is the most frequent mixed-cell type and usually produces AFP or hCG or both.

■ Other Combinations (20%)

In mixed-cell tumors, the prognosis becomes that of the most malignant element. Combinations with seminomas are treated as nonseminomatous tumors.

WORKUP

The usual presentation of testicular cancer is the incidental finding of a painless lump, nodule, swelling, or hardness in the testis of a young adult, which may be accompanied by a heavy sensation or dull ache in the lower abdomen. Occasionally, acute pain may occur because of rapid growth, resulting in hemorrhage and necrosis. Ten percent of patients will present with epididymitis. Up to 50% of patients will present with metastases, but only 10% will have symptoms of metastatic disease. Gynecomastia is seen in 5%.

History

Ask about a history of undescended testis, past trauma, chronic or repeated epididymitis, pain, weight loss, fever, or chills.

Physical Examination

The testis must be carefully palpated, starting with the normal side. A testis tumor is usually nontender and firm. A hydrocele can be transilluminated and drained with a needle to facilitate palpation. Check for supraclavicular nodes, gynecomastia, and groin, flank, or abdominal mass.

Laboratory Tests

Complete blood count (CBC), urinalysis, blood urea nitrogen (BUN), creatinine, β-hCG, and AFP are the recommended laboratory studies.

Imaging Studies

■ Ultrasound

Testicular ultrasound with color-flow Doppler is the mainstay for initial diagnosis of a testicular tumor to confirm physical findings or their absence. It should be performed in any patient in whom a testicular tumor is suspected. On occasion, surgical exploration will be necessary if a tumor cannot be ruled out by other means.

■ Computed Tomography Scan

Computed tomography (CT) scans of the abdomen and chest are the most effective imaging studies for metastatic evaluation. False-negative abdominal scans are not uncommon if nodal involvement measures less than 2 cm.

Metastatic Workup

After the diagnosis is confirmed by radical inguinal orchiectomy, further studies should include repeated markers for hCG (wait 1 week) and AFP (wait 4 weeks) and CT of the chest and abdomen. Note that staging accuracy is only 70% to 80%.

TREATMENT

Treatment strategies are based on the tumor's natural history (i.e., growth rate, pattern of spread, and radio- or chemosensitivity) and the clinical stage (i.e., nodal involvement and markers). A radical inguinal orchiectomy is the primary management for all solid testicular tumors. It confirms the diagnosis with pathologic identification of the histologic cell type and affords excellent local control. A retroperitoneal lymph node dissection (RPLND) has both staging and therapeutic value for selected patients with nonseminomatous tumors and spread to regional lymphatics. A limited nerve-sparing dissection can be used to preserve seminal emission in selected stage A patients with no gross disease on RPLND. Further treatment is based on the exquisite radiosensitivity of seminomas and the chemosensitivity of nonseminomas. Management of testicular cancer requires a team approach, including surgeon, medical oncologist, and radiation oncologist.

Seminomas

All patients receive a radical inguinal orchiectomy for diagnosis and local control. Because of the exquisite radiosensitivity of seminomas, external-beam radiotherapy continues to be the mainstay of treatment after orchiectomy for patients with low-volume retroperitoneal nodal involvement. Patients with high-volume retroperitoneal involvement or distant metastatic disease are managed with platinum-based chemotherapy.

■ Stage I: Tumor Confined to Scrotum

Radiation therapy (25 Gy) is delivered to periaortic and ipsilateral pelvic and inguinal lymph nodes. Supradiaphragmatic irradiation is not recommended. Five-year survival is 95%. Recent studies suggest that surveillance protocols may be offered to patients with stage I pure seminoma when the primary tumor is smaller than 6 cm, there is no vascular invasion, and β-hCG is normal. Patients whose disease relapses can usually be salvaged with chemotherapy.

■ Stage II: Tumor Confined to Retroperitoneum

Patients with stage II disease smaller than 5 cm confined to the retroperitoneum can be managed with 30 to 35 Gy of radiation, with a 5-year survival of approximately 80%. Patients with bulky retroperitoneal masses larger than 5 cm (N3) should receive primary platinum-based chemotherapy.

■ Stage III: Distant Metastatic Disease

Primary platinum-based chemotherapy is recommended.

Nonseminomas

Radiation therapy is ineffective against nonseminomas. Primary multidrug combination chemotherapy has been playing an ever-increasing role in nonseminomatous germ cell tumors, whereas the role of RPLNDs has been increasingly questioned. Approximately 50% to 70% of patients with nonseminomas will have metastatic disease at the time of diagnosis. The modified Einhorn regimen [cis-platinum, etoposide, and bleomycin (PEB)] is the preferred regimen for initial chemotherapy of patients with disseminated germ cell tumors. All patients receive an inguinal orchiectomy for diagnosis and local control. Close posttreatment follow-up is necessary to salvage those whose disease relapses (10%–20%). Salvage rate approaches 90%.

■ Stage I: Tumor Confined to Scrotum

Treatment of patients with clinical stage I (T1–T3, N0, M0) disease includes surveillance therapy, primary chemotherapy, or a staging and therapeutic RPLND followed by observation, or chemotherapy with BEP (two cycles) for those found to have nodal spread (25%). Because only 25% of stage I patients have pathologic disease found on RPLND, the surveillance option has been offered in appropriate cases in the hope of avoiding RPLND (see Surveillance Therapy).

■ Stage II: Tumor Confined to Retroperitoneum

Primary chemotherapy is increasingly used for patients with stage II disease. An RPLND is an option for patients with clinical evidence of low volume (N2) nodal disease followed by chemotherapy with BEP (two cycles).

■ Stage III: Distant Metastatic Disease

Patients with distant metastatic disease should have primary chemotherapy with PEB (three to four cycles). Use of RPLND for patients with bulky residual tumor after chemotherapy is unclear. Postchemotherapy masses are found to be fibrous tissue (40%), mature teratoma (40%), or persistent viable tumor (20%).

Salvage Chemotherapy

PEI (*cis*-platinum, etoposide, and ifosfamide) is the recommended regimen for relapse after standard PEB.

Complications of RPLND

Complications of RPLND include mortality of less than 1% and morbidity of 5% to 35%. Loss of seminal emission occurs in 75% of cases in which nerve-sparing technique is not used. Complication rates are greater with RPLND for postchemotherapy residual masses.

Surveillance Therapy

Surveillance therapy (e.g., radical orchiectomy followed by rigorous periodic reassessment, including tumor markers, chest radiograph, and CT scan every 2–3 months for the first 2 years) has been proposed for early-stage disease (pTis or pT1 and cN0) because of the complications of RPLND and the high salvage rates with chemotherapy and because only 25% of patients with clinical stage I disease have pathologic nodal spread. However, this should be undertaken with caution and only in highly controlled and structured follow-up programs. Surveillance programs report a 28% relapse rate; of these patients, 7% succumb to the disease.

Cancer of Urethra and Penis

CANCER OF URETHRA

Primary cancer of the urethra is an uncommon disease. It is the only urologic cancer that occurs more frequently in females than in males. Squamous cell carcinoma (SCC) represents the most common histologic type (80%); however, transitional cell carcinoma (15%), adenocarcinoma (5%), and, rarely, melanoma, also occur. Risk factors for the development of this tumor are chronic irritation and infection. Spread is primarily by direct extension to adjacent structures. Despite its tendency to remain localized, this is a disease with à poor prognosis, generally because it is found late in most cases. Lesions of the distal urethra have a better prognosis than do more proximal ones. A high index of suspicion is the key to diagnosis.

Cancer of Male Urethra

Urethral carcinoma in the male patient is associated with chronic inflammation, sexually transmitted disease, and strictures in the bulbomembranous portion of the urethra. Patients present with obstructive symptoms, recurrent strictures, a history of venereal disease, hematuria, or a sensation of a mass in the perineum. Spread is by direct extension to adjacent structures. Primary therapy is surgical excision.

Cancer of Female Urethra

Urethral carcinoma in the female patient is often found in the setting of urethral diverticula. Bleeding, dysuria, frequency, perineal pain, and dyspareunia are common presenting complaints. Most of these tumors are locally advanced when detected and involve the proximal urethra. Small distal tumors may respond well with radiation therapy or surgical excision alone.

Workup

The diagnosis is made by urethrography, urethroscopy, and repeated biopsy of the involved area. Staging is obtained by bimanual examination, magnetic resonance imaging, and computed tomography scan of chest, abdomen, and pelvis. In general, anterior or distal urethral tumors drain to the inguinal nodes, whereas posterior tumors drain to the pelvic nodes (i.e., obturator, presacral, and internal and external iliac nodes). Unlike those in cancer of the penis, clinically enlarged inguinal nodes usually imply metastatic disease and not benign inflammation. Tumor–node–metastasis (TNM) staging should be used.

Treatment

Unfortunately, the prognosis is poor for squamous carcinoma of the urethra despite radical surgery. Radiation and chemotherapy have little to offer these patients. Proximal tumors will usually require cystectomy and urethrectomy.

CANCER OF PENIS

Penile cancer is an uncommon disease (0.5% of malignancies in men in the United States) that occurs more frequently in older men. It has been associated with chronic inflammatory disease, venereal disease, human papilloma virus infection, and phimosis. Circumcision appears to be protective against the development of cancer of the penis. It occurs most frequently on the glans (50%), coronal sulcus, and prepuce (20%). More than 95% of cases are SCC. Hematogenous spread is rare; rather, an orderly spread via the lymphatics is the rule. Lymphatic spread is first to the superficial and deep inguinal nodes and then to the iliac nodes. The sentinel lymph node (located near the pubic tubercle and superficial epigastric vein) is believed to be the first point of lymphatic drainage for the penis. Patients often delay seeking medical attention and usually present with complaint of a nodular, ulcerative, or fungating penile lesion.

Carcinoma in Situ of the Penis

SCC in situ of the penis, also known as erythroplasia of Queyrat and Bowen's disease, can present as solitary painful or pruritic lesions of the penis. Erythroplasia of Queyrat is a velvety, erythematous lesion of the glans penis associated with burning and itching. Bowen's disease is a crusted or ulcerated plaque of the skin on the shaft of the penis. Diagnosis is made histologically, and treatment involves destroying the lesions with topical agents, cryotherapy, lasers, radiation, or surgery.

Workup

The definitive diagnosis of penile cancer is made only by histologic examination of a full-thickness biopsy. The tumor grade, depth of invasion, and configuration are important in planning management. Physical examination should include rectal and bimanual examination and inguinal palpation for adenopathy. A false-positive rate of up to 50% has been noted for clinically palpable inguinal nodes in penile cancer. Node enlargement secondary to inflammation is common; therefore, a short course of antibiotics (2–3 weeks) is recommended to help differentiate the true-positive nodes. Further staging includes chest radiograph, liver function tests, magnetic resonance imaging of the penis, ultrasound of inguinal nodes, and pelvic computed tomography scan. TNM staging should be used.

Treatment

■ Primary Neoplasm

The primary neoplasm is generally best treated by wide surgical excision leaving adequate tumor-free margins. Lesions confined to the prepuce can be managed with circumcision. Small Tis, Ta, and perhaps T1 lesions of the glans can be managed with laser therapy or Mohs micrographic surgery (MMS). Tumors confined to the glans or distal shaft will require partial amputation and reconstruction. Involvement of the proximal shaft or base of the penis necessitates total penectomy. In more advanced tumors, hemipelvectomy or hemicorporectomy is occasionally considered. Options for patients with carcinoma in situ (erythroplasia of Queyrat or Bowen's disease) include local excision, fulguration, radiation, lasers, or chemotherapy with topical (5%) 5-fluorouracil.

■ Inguinal Lymph Nodes

Clinically Positive Inguinal Examination

The presence of positive lymph node metastases portends a markedly worse prognosis. Palpable inguinal lymph nodes 4 to 6 weeks after control of the primary tumor and antibiotic therapy should be managed with lymphadenectomy. Bilateral inguinal lymphadenectomy is a therapeutic procedure conferring a 20% to 50% 5-year disease-free survival on patients with positive nodes compared with almost certain death if untreated.

Clinically Negative Inguinal Examination

Prophylactic inguinal lymphadenectomy is a highly morbid procedure with complications of thrombophlebitis, pulmonary embolism, wound infection, and lymphedema. However, clinical inguinal examination has a 2% to 25% false-negative rate. Patients with negative inguinal examinations should probably undergo lymphadenectomy in the setting of high-grade or invasive-stage (T2 or T3 N0M0) primary tumor. If superficial nodes are positive on frozen sections, then a complete therapeutic inguinal lymphadenectomy should be performed. Patients with low-grade, low-stage (Tis, Ta, T1 N0M0) tumors and negative inguinal examinations should undergo close surveillance for at least 2 to 3 years and be taught careful self-examination of the inguinal areas.

■ Pelvic Lymph Nodes

Pelvic lymphadenectomy is generally recommended only in healthy young individuals with positive inguinal nodes. The therapeutic benefit of pelvic node dissection has not been proven.

■ Advanced Inoperable Tumor (Jackson Stage IV)

Treatment is generally palliative chemotherapy or radiotherapy with aggressive combined-modality therapy, with chemotherapy and surgery reserved for the young patient.

VERRUCOUS CARCINOMA OF PENIS

Verrucous carcinoma of the penis is a peculiar slow-growing low-grade tumor that invades locally, destroying adjacent tissues by compression but shows no signs of malignant change on histologic examination and rarely metastasizes. It is sometimes classified as a variant of SCC that composes 5% to 15% of penile cancers. However, its correct classification is unclear. It is also referred to as a Buschke-Lowenstein tumor and giant condyloma acuminatum because of its similar gross appearance. Deep biopsies are required to make the histologic diagnosis and to examine for evidence of invasion, the hallmark of SCC. Wide surgical excision is the treatment of choice. Groin dissection is not necessary because lymph node metastases are rare. Radiotherapy is ineffective and should be avoided because it may transform the carcinoma into an aggressive metastasizing tumor.

Metabolic Disorders

NORMAL FLUID AND ELECTROLYTE REQUIREMENTS

Normal body homeostasis requires careful regulation of fluid volume and the concentration of electrolytes within the fluid. Volume regulation is primarily under the control of aldosterone, whereas tonicity is regulated by antidiuretic hormone (ADH). Volume has priority over tonicity when the protective mechanisms conflict.

Body Fluid Compartment	% Body Weight (kg)
Total body water	60
Intracellular fluid	40
Extracellular fluid	20
Blood (plasma 4% + RBCs 3%)	7

Maintenance Requirements

The normal daily maintenance requirements for fluid and electrolytes in an essentially healthy individual include the following.

Water	2 L/day
NaCl	75 mEq/day
K^+	40 mEq/day

Minimum daily water requirement for the body is based on the following needs:
- At least 600 mL urine is needed to keep the normal daily load of solutes in solution (1,000 mL in hypermetabolic, critically ill patients).
- Approximately 1,000 mL is needed to replace daily insensible water loss (i.e., from the respiratory tract and skin). These losses will increase with fever.

- Abnormal water losses include fluid loss in nasogastric suction, vomiting, diarrhea, fistula drainage, and third-space sequestration (e.g., ascites, bowel obstruction, retroperitoneal edema, and operative trauma).

Saline Solutions	Na mEq/L
Normal saline (NS; 0.9% NaCl)	154
Half-normal saline (0.45% NaCl)	77

Maintenance carbohydrate replacement of 100 to 150 g/day is necessary; 5% dextrose in water (D5W) contains 50 g/L glucose. A reasonable intravenous maintenance fluid for the uncomplicated hospitalized patient who is taking nothing by mouth (NPO) would be D5 0.5 NS with 20 mEq KCl per liter at 100 mL/hour. Replacement of any abnormal fluid losses should be added to this maintenance.

Abnormal Fluid-loss Replacements

- Gastric fluid is isotonic and high in K^+. Replacement: 0.5 NS with 40 mEq KCl/L.
- Fever or osmotic diuresis (as in diabetics or after hyperalimentation) results in hypotonic fluid loss (free water). Replacement: 0.5 NS.

Pediatric Intravenous Fluid Replacement	
Weight	mL/kg/day
First 10 kg (0–10)	100 +
Second 10 kg (10–20)	50 +
Each additional kilogram	20

ABNORMAL FLUID DISTURBANCES

Hypotonic Dehydration

Hypotonic dehydration occurs because of loss of isotonic fluid such as blood (hemorrhage), plasma (burns, pancreatitis, peritonitis), or gastrointestinal fluid (diarrhea) with secondary free-water retention, because of the increased ADH release with stress. *Treatment*—use normal saline for all fluid needs for a few days.

Hypotonic Overhydration

Hypotonic overhydration occurs because of inappropriate ADH secretion or acute renal failure. It most commonly occurs after the acute stress of surgery. *Treatment*—water restriction.

Hypertonic Dehydration

Hypertonic dehydration occurs because of excessive free-water loss as from the lungs (mechanical ventilation), perspiration (fever), osmotic diuresis (diabetes, hyperalimentation), or diabetes insipidus. *Treatment*—first correct hypovolemia with 0.5 NS, and then slowly correct tonicity with D5W (1 L D5W for each 3 mEq Na >140).

Transurethral Resection Syndrome

Transurethral resection (TUR) syndrome results from the sudden intravascular absorption of large volumes of hypotonic irrigating fluid, through the prostatic bed, during transurethral surgery. Clinical manifestations include hypertension, bradycardia, dyspnea, cyanosis, and mental confusion. *Treatment*—fluid restriction, diuretics (furosemide), and rarely hypertonic saline to restore tonicity (3% saline contains 513 mEq Na/L). The formula to calculate sodium deficit is

$$[\text{weight (kg)} \times 0.2] \times \Delta \text{serum Na (mEq/L)}$$

ELECTROLYTE DISORDERS

Hyperkalemia

The most common cause of hyperkalemia (K^+ >5.5 mEq/L) is acute oliguric renal failure. Other causes include potassium-sparing diuretics (e.g., spironolactone, triamterene, and amiloride), hypoaldosteronism, acidosis, rhabdomyolysis, and excessive potassium intake in the setting of renal insufficiency. Patients may demonstrate a generalized weakness, loss of deep tendon reflexes, irritability, and confusion. Electrocardiogram (ECG) changes, including peaked T waves, S-T depressions, and prolongation of the QRS, indicate significant hyperkalemia and may result in ventricular tachyarrhythmia or asystole.

■ **Treatment**

1. Shift potassium into cells with alkali or glucose (50 mEq $NaHCO_3$ IV bolus or 1 ampoule D50 glucose with 15 units of regular insulin).
2. Block effects of potassium on the heart with calcium (1 ampule calcium chloride or calcium gluconate given slowly).
3. Remove potassium from the body with potassium-binding resins (Kayexalate 10–30 g/100 mL as a retention enema for 15–20 minutes or 5–15 g PO qid).
4. Remove potassium from the body with dialysis (hemodialysis or peritoneal dialysis).
5. Eliminate underlying cause.

Hypokalemia

Hypokalemia (K^+ <3.5 mEq/L) most commonly results from increased potassium loss in gastrointestinal fluid (e.g., nasogastric suction, vomiting, diarrhea, and ureterosigmoidostomy) or urine [e.g., postobstructive diuresis, renal tubular acidosis (RTA), diuretics, hyperaldosteronism, and Cushing's syndrome]. Patients may demonstrate skeletal muscle weakness, ileus, abdominal distention, nausea, vomiting, and depressed sensorium. ECG changes include depressed T waves, sagging ST segments, and prominent U waves.

■ **Treatment**

1. Severe hypokalemia (K^+ <3.0 mEq/L) can be managed with intravenous KCl boluses not to exceed 20 mEq/hour or 240 mEq/day.
2. Oral potassium supplementation can be used for chronic potassium deficiencies.
3. Eliminate underlying cause.

Hyperchloremic Metabolic Acidosis

Hyperchloremic metabolic acidosis is a common complication of urinary diversions with intestines, especially when the urine remains in contact with the intestinal mucosa for prolonged periods as with ureterosigmoidostomies. Active chloride transport across the intestinal mucosa into the systemic circulation with an obligate cation is thought to be the mechanism. Hydrochloric acid or ammonium chloride accumulation or both result in the hyperchloremic metabolic acidosis.

■ **Treatment**

1. Restrict oral chloride and replace bicarbonate (e.g., sodium bicarbonate or potassium citrate).
2. Drain intestinal urinary reservoir.
3. Chlorpromazine (Thorazine) and nicotinic acid are drugs that block chloride transport via cyclic adenosine monophosphate (cAMP). Their use for treatment of chronic hyperchloremic metabolic acidosis has been suggested.

Hypercalcemia

Common causes of hypercalcemia include metastatic cancer to bone, hydrochlorothiazide therapy, and hyperparathyroidism. Patients may demonstrate weakness, somnolence, anorexia, polyuria, and coma. A history of stones, nephrocalcinosis, and hypophosphatemia suggests hyperparathyroidism as the etiology (measure serum parathyroid hormone). Patients with renal cell carcinoma may present with symptoms of hypercalcemia in fewer than 10% of cases. Production of a parathyroid-like hormone by the primary tumor has been suggested as a possible cause, in addition to hypercalcemia secondary to skeletal metastases with osteolysis.

■ **Treatment**

1. Initial therapy is to establish a sodium diuresis with intravenous saline administration followed by furosemide (Lasix).
2. Pamidronate (Aredia), 30 to 90 mg IV over a 24-hour period once will usually cause serum calcium to decrease within 12 to 24 hours and has been used for cases of severe hypercalcemia.

Hypocalcemia

Hypocalcemia is most commonly an artifact of hypoalbuminemia, which reduces the protein-bound fraction of total serum calcium. (Total calcium will decrease by 0.8 mg/dL for each decrement in serum albumin of 1 g/L.) Ionized calcium is normal, and the patient is asymptomatic in these cases. Causes of true hypocalcemia include hypoparathyroidism, hypomagnesemia, abnormalities in vitamin D metabolism, acute hyperphosphatemia or pancreatitis, blood transfusions, and osteoblastic metastases (e.g., breast, prostate, and lung). Acute hypocalcemia may be associated with tetany or latent tetany, as assessed by the Chvostek sign (tapping the facial nerve against the bone just anterior to the ear produces ipsilateral contraction of the facial muscles) or Trousseau's sign (induction of carpal spasm by occluding the brachial artery for 3 minutes) or both. Immediate treatment should be rendered because of the possibility of laryngeal spasms or seizures or both.

■ Treatment

1. Intravenous calcium gluconate is appropriate initial therapy for patients with tetany or latent tetany.
2. Chronic hypocalcemia is managed with oral calcium and vitamin D supplementation. (Remember first to reduce hyperphosphatemia in patients with renal failure.)

Hypermagnesemia

Hypermagnesemia rarely occurs in the setting of normal renal function. It can occur, however, when using Suby's solution G or magnesium carbonate (Renacidin) for irrigation of the urinary system to dissolve stones. The impaired neuromuscular transmission that results can produce mental confusion, drowsiness, muscular paralysis, and occasionally coma.

■ Treatment

1. A sodium diuresis with saline and furosemide (Lasix) is usually effective therapy.
2. When symptoms are severe, emergency treatment with calcium gluconate should be undertaken, followed by hemodialysis if the patient has decreased renal function.

RENAL TUBULAR ACIDOSIS

RTA refers to a disorder of urinary acidification. The inability to excrete acid into the urine results in a systemic metabolic acidosis and concurrent elevated serum chloride. The higher urinary pH increases urine phosphate levels. Three major types of renal tubular acidosis are recognized: types I, II, and IV. Type III RTA is now considered a variant of type I.

Type I Renal Tubular Acidosis (Distal)

Classic RTA is caused by an inability of the distal tubule to secrete hydrogen ion into the urine. Urinary wasting of calcium, phosphorus, and potassium also is noted in this syndrome. Nephrocalcinosis or nephrolithiasis will occur in about 70% of patients. The diagnosis is made in the setting of a systemic acidosis (serum bicarbonate <20 mEq/L) with an inappropriately high urinary pH (>5.5). In adults, the disorder is persistent and is found predominantly in women, whereas the infantile form is transient but can result in significant growth impairment. *Treatment*—fluid and electrolyte replacement with potassium citrate.

Type II Renal Tubular Acidosis (Proximal)

Type II RTA is caused by a defect in the reabsorption of filtered bicarbonate in the proximal tubule. Initially, massive bicarbonaturia is found; however, as the plasma bicarbonate level decreases with consequent worsening systemic acidosis, the filtered load of bicarbonate also decreases, resulting in disappearance of bicarbonaturia and normal urinary pH. It is often associated with other proximal tubular defects such as Fanconi's syndrome, hereditary fructose intolerance, Wilson's disease, or multiple myeloma. However, vitamin D deficiency secondary to intestinal malabsorption is the most common cause in adults. Nephrolithiasis does not occur. *Treatment*—vitamin D therapy will correct the acidification defect in patients with vitamin D deficiency; otherwise therapy is directed at treating the acidosis with alkali (e.g., potassium citrate or bicarbonate).

Type IV Renal Tubular Acidosis

Type IV hyperkalemic RTA occurs because of a defect in aldosterone-dependent potassium ion secretion. It most frequently is noted in elderly diabetics with hyporeninemic hypoaldosteronism. Mineralocorticoid replacement (fludrocortisone 0.1 mg/day) will reverse hyperkalemia and acidosis.

■ Renal Tubular Acidosis Syndromes			
	Type I	Type II	Type IV
Site	Distal	Proximal	Distal
Defect	H^+ secretion	HCO_3 reabsorption	Aldosterone
Serum K^+	Low	Low	High
Other	Stones	Fanconi's syndrome	

Obstructive Uropathy

Obstruction to urine flow can occur anywhere in the urinary tract. Proximal to the obstruction, pressures within the collecting system and renal tubules will increase. Ultimately renal injury will result because of cellular atrophy and necrosis if the obstruction to urine flow is not relieved. Acute obstruction will produce distention of the bladder, ureter, or renal pelvis that is generally associated with pain. However, a slowly progressing obstruction can result in massive dilatation of the collecting system with no clinical symptoms. Recovery of some renal function can generally be expected in cases of complete unilateral ureteral obstruction if flow is restored within 6 weeks.

CAUSES OF OBSTRUCTION

The most frequent causes of obstruction in adult men are stones, benign prostatic hyperplasia, prostate cancer, ureteropelvic junction (UPJ) obstruction, and ureteral strictures, whereas in women, the most frequent causes are pregnancy, stones, UPJ obstruction, pelvic malignancies, and surgical trauma to the ureters. In children, UPJ obstruction, ureterovesical junction obstruction (e.g., ectopic ureters), ureteroceles, urethral valves, and stones are most frequently responsible for urinary obstruction.

Causes of obstruction can be more systematically evaluated by location.

■ Bladder Outlet Obstruction	
Mechanical	Functional
Benign prostatic hyperplasia	Neurogenic (detrusor-sphincter dyssynergia)
Urethral stricture	Pharmacologic
Bladder neck contracture	
Posterior urethral valves	
Ureteroceles	
Urethral stone	
Foreign body	

■ Ureteral Obstruction	
Intrinsic Obstruction	**Extrinsic Obstruction**
Stones	Pregnancy
Tumors	Tumor
Strictures	Retroperitoneal fibrosis
(tuberculosis, radiation, previous	Crossing blood vessel to lower pole of
instrumentation)	kidney (UPJ)
Adynamic segment at UPJ	Retrocaval ureter
	Pelvic lipomatosis
	Iatrogenic ligature
UPJ, ureteropelvic junction.	

DIAGNOSIS

The diagnosis of lower urinary tract obstruction must always be the first consideration in the patient who presents with oligo-anuria. The simple passage of a urethral catheter or percutaneous suprapubic catheter is both diagnostic and therapeutic. Upper urinary tract obstruction will require more specialized diagnostic techniques.

Renal Ultrasound

Renal ultrasound is a quick, noninvasive method of identifying upper-tract obstruction and can be used in the setting of an elevated creatinine level. Occasionally upper-tract obstruction may not cause significant hydronephrosis and may result in a false negative renal ultrasound.

Excretory Urography

An intravenous urogram is the method of choice for demonstrating upper-tract obstruction in the patient with a normal serum creatinine level. It gives anatomic insight into the location and etiology of the obstruction. Obstruction is evident by a prolonged nephrogram, delayed calyceal filling, and dilatation of the collecting system proximal to the site of obstruction. With severe obstruction, no function may be seen; however, it is important to obtain delayed films for at least several hours to look for delayed excretion.

Retrograde and Anterograde Pyelography

The retrograde injection of contrast up the ureter during cystoscopy is the gold standard for ruling out ureteral obstruction. It can define the lowermost extent of any ureteral obstruction and can be used in the setting of renal failure or contrast hypersensitivity. Anterograde injection of contrast via a percutaneous nephrostomy also is an option under these circumstances.

Nuclear Renograms

Mercaptoacetylglycine (MAG3) or diethylenetriaminepentaacetate (DTPA) renal scans are useful in the evaluation of the patient with suspected obstruction. They can be used even in the setting of contrast hypersensitivity or mildly impaired renal function. MAG3 or hippuran scans are more useful in the setting of moderate renal failure. With the addition of a diuretic such as furosemide (Lasix), renal scans can usually differentiate partial obstructions and dilated, but unobstructed, systems (e.g., megacalyces or megaureter).

Pressure/Flow Perfusion: The Whitaker Test

Normal pressure differential between the renal pelvis and bladder during a constant-flow infusion of the renal pelvis at 10 mL/min should be less than15 cm H_2O. Pressures of more than 22 cm H_2O suggest obstruction.

MANAGEMENT

Relief of urinary tract obstruction should be obtained expeditiously. Prospects for recovery of function are directly related to degree and duration of the obstruction. Temporary catheter drainage of the upper or lower urinary tract should be provided until definitive repair can be performed. The kidney's potential for recovery after long-standing obstruction also can be determined before undertaking a major surgical procedure by providing temporary catheter drainage and monitoring creatinine clearance.

Postobstructive Diuresis

After the relief of long-standing urinary tract obstruction with elevated blood urea nitrogen (BUN) and creatinine, a physiologic diuresis can be expected. This is usually a self-limiting nephropathy, which can be managed with proper fluid and electrolyte replacement. Patients with very high BUN and creatinine levels or urine output greater than 200 mL/hour for 2 consecutive hours are at increased risk of a pathologic diuresis, which will require monitoring and management. Occasionally, it can lead to severe hypovolemia and even shock. Three different physiologic types of diuresis are described.

■ Types of Diuresis

Urea Diuresis

Urea diuresis is most common and occurs secondary to the osmotic load of the urea retained during obstruction. The excretion of excess urea and water after relief of obstruction is self-limiting, lasting only 24 to 48 hours, and requires little attention.

Salt Diuresis

Salt diuresis is the second most common variety. The excess total body salt and water that is retained during obstruction is generally excreted in a self-limiting fashion until a normovolemic state is reached. However, a salt-and-water diuresis may occasionally continue in a pathologic manner well after normal fluid balance has been established. It is therefore important to monitor and replace fluid and electrolytes carefully during a salt diuresis to avoid severe dehydration and salt depletion.

Water Diuresis

Water diuresis occurs as a self-limited nephrogenic diabetes insipidus in the absence of an expanded total body water. This is believed to occur rarely.

■ Diagnosis

Measure urine sodium, potassium, and osmolarity. The osmolarity should approximate twice the urine sodium and urine potassium (in mEq/L) plus the urea.

$$\text{Urea Diuresis} \leftrightarrow 2 \times (U_{Na} + U_K) = <(\tfrac{1}{2}) \text{ Osmolarity}$$

$$\text{Salt Diuresis} \leftrightarrow 2 \times (U_{Na} + U_K) = >(\tfrac{1}{2}) \text{ Osmolarity}$$

■ Treatment

A urea diuresis is generally self-limiting and will cease when the BUN returns to normal. Monitoring output and electrolytes is usually sufficient. A salt diuresis, conversely, will require more aggressive management because of the potential for prolonged duration of more than 72 hours. Careful monitoring of input and output, serum and urine electrolytes, and central venous pressures is appropriate. If the diuresis persists after the patient's edema fluid has been excreted, then replacement therapy should be started. Intravenous replacement should approximate the electrolyte concentration of the urine, giving 0.5 mL for each milliliter of urine on an hourly basis. Overzealous fluid replacement can result in perpetuation of a self-limiting salt diuresis.

IDIOPATHIC CAUSES OF OBSTRUCTION

Retroperitoneal Fibrosis

Retroperitoneal fibrosis is a chronic inflammatory process of unknown etiology in most cases. It produces a fibrotic retroperitoneal mass that is typically situated in the region between the renal pedicles and the sacral promontory. As the process progresses, it easily compresses the ureters as it drags them medially, causing obstructive uropathy and hydroureteronephrosis above the level of the sacral promontory. It affects both male and female patients in a 2:1 ratio, usually in the fifth and sixth decades. Its etiology is unknown in the vast majority of cases; however, some conditions associated with its occurrence include the use of certain drugs (methysergide, methyldopa, hydralazine, β-blockers, etc.), chemicals (Avitene, talcum powder), inflammatory processes [perianeurysmal inflammation, chronic inflammatory bowel disease, gonococcal infection (GC), tuberculosis, syphilis], radiation injury, and malignancies.

■ Diagnosis

Pain is the most frequent presenting complaint; it is typically a dull ache in the lower back, flank, or abdomen that radiates to both lower quadrants, the umbilicus, or testicles. The excretory intravenous urogram will demonstrate medial deviation of the middle third of the ureter with proximal hydroureteronephrosis secondary to extrinsic ureteral compression. Computed tomography scan may show a dense retroperitoneal mass anterior to the great vessels. Histologic diagnosis by biopsy must be performed to rule out malignancy.

■ Treatment

Initial management entails decompression of the upper urinary tract with indwelling ureteral stents or percutaneous nephrostomy tubes. Definitive management will require abdominal exploration for a diagnostic biopsy and ureteral lysis and lateralization or intraperitonealization of the ureters. A course of corticosteroid therapy (prednisone) has been advocated by some to retard progression of the disease and to prevent its recurrence.

Pelvic Lipomatosis

Pelvic lipomatosis is a rare proliferative process of unknown etiology that involves the mature fat of the pelvic retroperitoneum. It occurs primarily in overweight men (predominantly black) in the third to sixth decades and is usually discovered incidentally, with no presenting symptoms. The diagnosis is made by the typical radiolucency of lipomatous tissue surrounding the bladder on kidney, ureter, and bladder (KUB) films. The intravenous urogram usually demonstrates normal upper tract and vertical elongation of the bladder with a pear or teardrop shape. On occasion, ureteral obstruction with hydroureteronephrosis has been noted. A computed tomography scan is ideal for the diagnosis. Treatment is generally conservative and consists of diet control and massive weight reduction.

30 Renal Failure

ACUTE RENAL FAILURE

Acute renal failure (ARF) is a condition of abrupt deterioration in renal function as evidenced by increasing blood urea nitrogen (BUN) and creatinine and usually decreased urine output. Approximately half of all cases occur in the surgical setting, and early recognition can minimize the extent of renal injury. The following is a brief review of the three major classifications of acute renal failure.

Prerenal

Prerenal azotemia is the direct result of inadequate renal perfusion. If the reason for poor perfusion can be rapidly reversed, resolution of the problem can usually be expected. However, prolonged low-flow states can produce an intrinsic ischemic injury to the kidney [i.e., acute tubular necrosis (ATN)].

■ Causes of Prerenal Azotemia

1. Volume depletion (hemorrhage, dehydration)
2. Low cardiac output (congestive heart failure, cardiogenic shock, tamponade)
3. Renal artery (stenosis, occlusion, vasoconstriction)
4. Systemic vasodilatation (sepsis, anaphylaxis, overdose)

Postrenal

Obstruction to urine flow can occur anywhere in the urinary tract. Proximal to the obstruction, pressures within the collecting system and renal tubules will increase. Ultimately renal injury will result because of cellular atrophy and necrosis if the obstruction to urine flow is not relieved. Recovery of some renal function can generally be expected in cases of complete unilateral ureteral obstruction if flow is restored within 6 weeks.

■ **Causes of Urinary Obstruction**

1. Bladder outlet (benign prostatic hyperplasia, strictures, bladder-neck contracture, stones, foreign body, tumor, blood clots, etc.)
2. Ureters (stones, intrinsic and extrinsic tumors, retroperitoneal fibrosis, papillary necrosis, ureteropelvic junction obstruction)

Intrarenal

Acute parenchymal renal failure is the result of tubular cell damage from hypoperfusion, nephrotoxic injury, or an inflammatory process.

■ **Causes of Intrinsic Parenchymal Renal Disease**

- ATN can be conveniently divided into three phases: (a) onset, (b) oliguric, and (c) postoliguric. The oliguric period (urine output <500 mL/24 hours) typically lasts 10 to 14 days; however, it may be as brief as 2 days or as long as 6 to 8 weeks. A nonoliguric ATN can occur particularly when secondary to nephrotoxic injury such as aminoglycosides or radiographic contrast agents. Causes of ATN include the following:
  1. Ischemic injury from renal hypoperfusion (hypotensive episodes, cardiogenic or septic shock, etc.) is the most common cause of ATN in hospitalized patients.
  2. Nephrotoxins [aminoglycosides, anesthetics, iodinated contrast media, nonsteroidal antiinflammatory drugs (NSAIDs)].
  3. Hemoglobinuria or myoglobinuria (intravascular hemolysis or rhabdomyolysis).
- Acute glomerular nephritis—urinalysis is important [proteinuria, hematuria, and red blood cell (RBC) casts].
- Acute interstitial nephritis—sterile pyuria, white blood cell (WBC) casts, and eosinophiluria, most often caused by drugs [NSAIDs, percutaneous nephrostolithotomy (PCN), sulfonamides, cimetidine, allopurinol, ciprofloxacin].

Evaluation of Acute Renal Failure

The workup of a patient with sudden elevation of BUN and creatinine with or without decreased urine output requires a prompt, systematic approach to exclude any reversible pathophysiologic states and to remove any potentially nephrotoxic agents. Prerenal and postrenal causes must be excluded before diagnosing intrinsic renal disease.

■ Renal Hypoperfusion

Evaluate Circulatory System

Measure heart rate, blood pressure, postural hypotension, jugular venous distention, central venous pressures, and cardiac output (Swan-Ganz catheter if necessary), and listen to the chest for evidence of heart failure.

Check Volume Status

Assess weights, input/output records, skin turgor, mucous membranes, recent surgery, gastrointestinal bleeding, urine specific gravity (usually >1.015–1.020) and/or osmolality, BUN/creatinine ratio (>20:1), spot urine sodium (<5 mEq/L), and fractional excretion of sodium.

Urinalysis

Urinalysis is typically unremarkable.

Evaluate Renal Vasculature

Obtain diethylene triamine pentaacetate (DTPA) renal scan, arteriography, or venography.

■ Urinary Obstruction

Bladder Outlet

Place a Foley catheter or irrigate existing catheter.

Upper Tracts

Perform renal ultrasound or stone protocol computed tomography (CT) and retrograde urograms.

■ Intrinsic Renal Injury

Urinalysis

The urinary sediment will typically show renal tubular cell casts during the early stages of ATN. Urine specific gravity is usually fixed at 1.010 to 1.012, and the urinary sodium concentration is greater than 30 to 40 mEq/L. Proteinuria is observed with glomerular disease and to a lesser extent with interstitial disease.

Ischemia

Look for periods of hypotension (e.g., recent surgery or septic or cardiogenic shock).

Nephrotoxins

Carefully check for medications that can cause ATN (e.g., aminoglycoside, antibiotics, recent radiographic contrast studies) or interstitial nephritis [e.g., sulfa drugs, penicillin, furosemide, hydrochlorothiazide (HCTZ), dilantin] or medications that exacerbate prerenal azotemia (e.g., prostaglandin inhibitors, NSAIDs).

Hemoglobinuria or Myoglobinuria
Look for recent trauma, burns, or surgery.

Management of Acute Renal Failure

1. Reverse any pathophysiologic states—restore volume, support blood pressure, and treat sepsis or cardiac failure.
2. Relieve any urinary obstruction—ensure adequate drainage of urinary tract as needed (e.g., Foley catheter, suprapubic tube, ureteral stents, or nephrostomy tubes). Monitor and treat post-obstructive diuresis.
3. Remove any nephrotoxic agents; stop any nephrotoxic drugs (i.e., change antibiotics as needed, discontinue NSAIDs).
4. Restrict sodium, potassium, and fluid intake.
5. Minimize risk of infectious complications—avoid use of Foley catheters or central venous lines if possible.
6. Convert to nonoliguria if possible—persistent oliguria after correction of pre- and postrenal causes is strong evidence of intrinsic renal failure. A trial of furosemide or an osmotic diuretic may convert the patient from oliguric to nonoliguric renal failure. This will make patient management easier and decrease the frequency and duration of dialysis during the recovery phase.
7. Support with dialysis as needed.

■ Indications for Dialysis in Acute Renal Failure

1. Volume overload manifested by pulmonary edema and decreased pO_2 unresponsive to diuretics
2. Hyperkalemia or marked acidosis or both in the setting of volume overload
3. Uremic manifestations (e.g., change in mental status, seizures, cardiac complications, gastrointestinal bleeding)
4. BUN greater than 100 or creatinine greater than 10 without clear prospects for early recovery

CHRONIC RENAL FAILURE

Etiology

Chronic renal failure (CRF) is caused by a spectrum of diseases resulting in progressive irreversible loss of functioning nephrons, ultimately leading to end-stage renal disease (ESRD) requiring dialysis or transplantation if not halted. The most common etiologies are diabetes mellitus, hypertension, primary and secondary glomerular diseases, hereditary renal disease, obstructive uropathy, chronic infection, and interstitial nephritis.

Manifestations

Uremic symptoms of CRF rarely occur until the glomerular filtration rate (GFR) is less than 25 mL/minute (25% of normal) or the serum creatinine is more than 3 to 4 mg/dL. A wide variety of systemic symptoms involving all organ systems can be seen. This multisystem involvement can make management of these patients quite difficult.

■ Metabolic

Hyperphosphatemia

Hyperphosphatemia is an early and cardinal manifestation of ESRD and is in itself responsible for many secondary stigmata of the disease. Some evidence suggests that reducing dietary phosphate intake can slow progression of CRF.

Hyperkalemia

Hyperkalemia is generally not a problem in CRF until the GFR decreases to less than 5 mL/minute.

Acidosis

A positive anion-gap metabolic acidosis occurs because of the impaired ability of the kidneys to produce ammonia (if GFR is <25 mL/minute).

■ Gastrointestinal

Gastrointestinal involvement includes nausea, vomiting, anorexia, a metallic taste, uremic stomatitis, glossitis, esophagitis, gastritis, peptic ulcer disease from gastric hypersecretion, colitis, diverticulosis, constipation, and fecal impaction. Upper and lower gastrointestinal bleeding is a not uncommon complication.

■ Hematologic

A normochromic normocytic anemia secondary to marrow suppression and decreased renal erythropoietin occurs when the BUN exceeds 60 to 80 mg/dL or the creatinine increases to greater than 2 to 3 mg/dL. Thrombocytopenia and platelet dysfunction also occur. Patients undergoing surgery (especially transurethral resection of the prostate) are at increased risk for bleeding complications. Dialysis helps to reverse these problems partially.

■ Neurologic

Uremic peripheral neuropathy and encephalopathy can be controlled with adequate dialysis or transplantation.

■ Cardiovascular

CRF is associated with an increased incidence and severity of atherosclerosis. Derangements in protein and lipid metabolism with hypertriglyceridemia and prolonged hypertension are considered to be major factors involved.

■ Endocrine Dysfunction

Renal Osteodystrophy

The abnormal bone metabolism found in CRF has a multifactorial origin. First, hyperphosphatemia, due to reduced GFR, directly reduces serum ionized calcium. This reduction stimulates parathyroid hormone (PTH) secretion (secondary hyperparathyroidism) and consequent bone resorption. Second, loss of renal parenchyma results in decreased renal conversion of 25-hydroxy-D_3 to the active 1,25-dihydroxy-D_3. Additionally, hyperphosphatemia inhibits this synthesis. Third, chronic metabolic acidosis is buffered by bone with consequent demineralization. Patients will have bone pain, particularly arthralgias, and pleuritic chest-wall pain. Management is directed toward control of hyperphosphatemia by limiting dietary intake of phosphorus to less than 1 g/day. Only after serum phosphorus levels have been reduced can supplemental calcium and the active metabolite of vitamin D [1,25-dihydroxycholecalciferol (Rocaltrol)] be given. Parathyroidectomy is rarely necessary.

Glucose Intolerance

Glucose intolerance secondary to peripheral insulin resistance is common in CRF and generally does not require treatment.

Sexual Dysfunction

Sexual dysfunction is a prominent component of renal failure. Loss of libido and development of impotence occurs in more than 50% of patients. Serum testosterone levels are usually low. Women commonly have loss of libido with dysmenorrhea and amenorrhea.

Management

The general management of patients with CRF centers on slowing the progression of functional renal deterioration. No effective treatment exists for most glomerulopathies, except for minimal-change disease, which often responds to steroids. Any reversible or controllable factors must be addressed, such as hypertension, obstructive uropathy, or infections. Dietary measures involving control of protein and phosphorus intake have been shown to be beneficial by decreasing the remnant nephron hyperfiltration and glomerular hypertension. Once the GFR deteriorates to levels that produce significant symptoms of ESRD (e.g., creatinine clearance <5 mL/minute), then dialysis or transplantation becomes the only option. However, any residual renal function, even a clearance of 2 to 5 mL/minute, can be important in modifying the urgency, duration, and frequency of dialysis.

DIALYSIS

Fortunately most symptomatic manifestations of CRF and ESRD are greatly improved by dialysis.

Hemodialysis

■ Principles of Hemodialysis

The basic elements of hemodialysis involve blood flow on one side of a semipermeable membrane and the dialysate, an osmotically balanced solution of electrolytes and glucose in water, on the other side of the membrane. Primarily small-molecular-weight molecules passively diffuse down concentration gradients across the membrane, which accounts for the clearance effect. Additionally, a positive blood pressure on one side of the membrane allows mass fluid transfer known as ultrafiltration. By these two mechanisms of clearance and ultrafiltration, the dialyzer can remove toxic waste products from the blood and maintain fluid homeostasis. Serum electrolytes can be kept within limits by carefully adjusting their concentration in the dialysate. The patient's fluid status can be controlled by manipulating the positive and negative transmembrane pressures to remove just as much volume as needed.

■ Vascular Access

Maintenance of proper access for hemodialysis can be a major challenge for both the surgeon and the patient. The various options available must be understood.

Temporary Access

Temporary access is often necessary for immediate urgent dialysis of patients with life-threatening situations.

1. *Percutaneous transvenous catheters* using the Seldinger technique and an internal jugular or femoral approach is generally the preferred method. A dual-lumen coaxial catheter with separate inflow and outflow works well. Patency is maintained by continuous or intermittent flushing with heparinized saline. These catheters can be maintained for 2 to 3 weeks in the internal jugular vein.

2. *External Scribner shunt*—this is still occasionally used when efficient high-flow dialysis is needed or when the percutaneous transvenous approach is contraindicated.

Maintenance Access

Maintenance access is provided by a subcutaneous arteriovenous (AV) fistula (Cimino) with endogenous vein or prosthetic graft material. External shunts (Scribner) have been generally abandoned for long-term access.

1. *Endogenous AV fistula*—the classic choice is the endogenous radial-cephalic side-to-side AV fistula, described by Cimino in 1966, in the nondominant arm. Three-year patency rates of almost 80% have been reported. Failure is usually from thrombosis or aneurysms.

2. *Prosthetic AV fistula*—use of a vascular prosthesis [6-mm polytetrafluoroethylene (PTFE)] is necessary in patients without suitable endogenous veins available. Infection is the most common cause of failure.

■ Maintenance Dialysis

In general, the predialysis BUN ranges between 50 and 200 mg/dL, and the creatinine, from 5 to 25 mg/dL, and both can be expected to be reduced by about 50% during dialysis. A typical stable patient will require dialysis 3 times per week for a total of 12 to 18 hours.

■ Complications of Hemodialysis

Hypotension

Patients are generally kept as close to dry weight as possible. The potential for major fluid shifts must be strictly controlled.

Systemic Heparinization

Systemic heparinization can result in major bleeding complications, particularly gastrointestinal. Do not perform diagnostic or therapeutic procedures on recently dialyzed patients (e.g., lumbar puncture).

Rapid Osmotic Changes

Rapid osmotic changes can produce significant central nervous system dysfunction from cerebral edema (referred to as the dialysis disequilibrium syndrome).

Hemolysis

Hemolysis can result from a failure to maintain proper dialysate osmolarity.

Membrane Rupture

Membrane rupture within the dialyzer can result in significant blood loss if not recognized promptly.

Air Embolus

Air embolus can occur when administering medications or solutions into the arterial line.

Peritoneal Dialysis

The principles of peritoneal dialysis are similar to those of hemodialysis. Dialysate is placed within the peritoneal cavity for specific lengths of time (dwell time), and the peritoneum acts as the semipermeable membrane separating the dialysate and blood. It can be performed in the short term by using a simple straight peritoneal catheter or on a long-term basis, which requires placement of a Tenckhoff catheter. An advantage of peritoneal dialysis is that it can provide more even control of hyperkalemia without the hyperdynamic effects of hemodialysis. Peritonitis is the most common complication of peritoneal dialysis.

▪ Indications for Peritoneal Dialysis

1. Patients without vascular access
2. Patients with contraindications for heparinization (e.g., bleeding diathesis)
3. Patients with unstable coronary artery disease or low ejection fractions who may not tolerate hypotensive episodes

▪ Contraindications for Peritoneal Dialysis

1. Recent abdominal surgery
2. Compromised respiratory function

▪ Long-term Peritoneal Dialysis

Prolonged peritoneal dialysis is performed either intermittently with 10- to 14-hour dwell times, three times per week, or almost continuously by the patient changing the dialysate four or five times per day, 7 days/week—continuous ambulatory peritoneal dialysis (CAPD).

KIDNEY TRANSPLANTATION

Renal transplantation is clearly the preferred treatment for patients with permanent renal failure (GFR, <10 mL/minute, or serum creatinine, >8 mg/dL). It provides significantly longer survival over dialysis and a better quality of life. Because of the increasing numbers of patients requiring transplantation and the long waits for cadaveric kidneys, living related-donor renal transplantation is increasing. Living related donors have a better probability of graft survival and can allow patients to have preemptive renal transplantation before ever needing to go on dialysis.

Recipient Selection

▪ Contraindications to Transplantation
1. Active infection
2. Recent malignant disease
3. Active glomerulonephritis
4. Presensitization to donor class I human leukocyte antigen (HLA) antigens

▪ Pretransplant Blood Transfusions
Data have paradoxically shown that nontransfused patients have the highest risk of graft failure and that performing up to 14 transfusions before transplantation appears to impart a dose-related increase in cadaveric graft survival.

Donor Selection

▪ Living Related Donors
Living related and unrelated donors are an increasing source of kidney transplants in the United States because of superior graft survival and a shortage of cadaveric kidneys. Donors are expected to be in perfect physical and mental health with negative blood and tissue cross-matches. Compatibility by mixed lymphocyte culture is demonstrated by negative HLA antigenic stimulation. Graft success can be improved between responders by using donor-specific transfusions.

■ Cadaver Donors

Cadaver donors are generally persons between ages 2 and 60 years without evidence of significant hypertension, atherosclerosis, renal disease, malignancy, or infection. Blood and urine cultures should be negative, with creatinine less than 2 mg/dL, and hepatitis B antigen (HBsAg) negative. The heart must be pumping, and no longer than 10 minutes of warm ischemia should exist. Blood pressure (systolic blood pressure >100 mm Hg) and urine output (>100 mL/hour) should be maintained by volume expansion, diuretics, and, if necessary, vasopressors as needed (dopamine preferred). After removal, kidneys are flushed with ice-cold Collins' solution and stored in ice slush (for 24–48 hours) or preserved by pulsatile perfusion (for 48–72 hours).

Tissue Matching

A single chromosomal complex of closely linked genes codes for a group of antigens that have been shown to represent the strongest immunologic barrier to transplantation. These major histocompatibility antigens are the product of two sets of HLA genes on homologous paired chromosomes, one set or haplotype from each parent. The HLA gene products (cell-surface antigens) from each haplotype are classified as class I serologically defined HLA-A, -B, and -C and the class II HLA-DR (D-related) antigens, the major initiator of the mixed lymphocyte reaction (MLR). The paternal and maternal alleles from each of the four HLA loci are expressed in a codominant fashion. Matching for major HLA antigens among closely related living donors has been shown to predict results superior to those with cadaveric donors because of compatibility among other less important gene products of the major histocompatibility complex (MHC) region. HLA type matching for cadaveric transplants is less successful because of the greater variation among the minor transplantation antigens, and its usefulness has been questioned. However, many centers still attempt to use a four-antigen match, referring to two A and two B locus antigen matching, in addition to testing for preexisting anti-HLA antibodies by the lymphocytotoxic cross-match. This improves the statistical probability of identical HLA-C and -D locus antigens, but it is not a certainty. The MLR test for HLA-DR antigens takes 6 to 8 days and is therefore not clinically useful for cadaveric transplants. Serologic typing for class II antigens can provide an approximation of mixed lymphocyte culture reactivity.

Living related transplants between HLA identical siblings (two-haplotype match) yield the highest 1-year graft survival (up to 90%), followed next by HLA semi-identical (one-haplotype match).

The ABO (H) blood group antigens are expressed on vascular endothelium and therefore must be matched for renal transplantation. However, Rh antigens are not expressed on nucleated cells and need not be of concern.

Immunosuppression

The allograft response is directed primarily against mismatched HI.A antigens and is T cell dependent. Class II HLA alloantigens activate helper T lymphocytes, resulting in release of macrophage-stimulating lymphokine (MSL) and expression of interleukin-1 (IL-1) and -2 (IL-2) receptors on helper T cells. Class I HLA alloantigens activate cytotoxic T lymphocytes to form IL-2 receptors. Stimulated macrophages release IL-1, which in turn causes the release of IL-2 from helper T cells. It is the IL-2 that then causes the specific clonal proliferation of activated helper and cytotoxic T cells. Immunosuppressive therapies are directed toward interfering with one or more of these steps in the allograft response.

▦ Corticosteroids

Corticosteroids inhibit IL-2–dependent T-cell proliferation by preventing monocytes from releasing IL-1 that is necessary for release of IL-2. They also have an inhibitory effect on neutrophilic inflammatory response.

▦ Azathioprine (Imuran)

Azathioprine is a mainstay of therapy for acute rejection and functions by inhibiting the multiplication of rapidly dividing immunologically competent lymphoid cells. Its major toxic side effect, myelosuppression, is best guarded against by monitoring the peripheral leukocyte count.

▦ Mycophenolate Mofetil (CellCept)

Mycophenolate is a product of *Penicillium* species, and its mode of action is similar to that of azathioprine. Its main advantage over azathioprine is less bone marrow suppression.

▦ Cyclosporine (Sandimmune or Neoral)

Cyclosporine (CsA) acts primarily by the specific and reversible inhibition of activated T-cell proliferation and by blocking the release of IL-2 by activated helper T cells. It has significant side effects including potent nephrotoxicity and dose-dependent hepatotoxicity, hirsutism, and tremors. It is eliminated primarily by the liver with a mean half-life of 19 hours and is *not* dialyzable. Peak plasma concentrations are reached in approximately 3.5 hours. Trough levels should be maintained between 100 and 200 ng/mL and checked two or three times per week for the first 2 weeks. Avoid use of other potentially nephrotoxic drugs, such as furosemide and aminoglycosides.

▪ Tacrolimus

Tacrolimus is a macrolide antibiotic similar to CsA in its activity. It can cause nephrotoxicity, neurotoxicity, and a drug-induced diabetes mellitus. It is used primarily in women because of the lack of associated hirsutism.

▪ Antithymocyte γ-Globulin

Antithymocyte γ-globulin (ATG) is the pooled polyclonal globulin fraction of sera from horses immunized to human thymocytes (nonspecific antibodies are absorbed out). ATG has shown itself to be a potent suppressor of cell-mediated immunity and allograft response. It is used either for early immunosuppression or to treat acute rejection. Anaphylactoid responses occur, and it is given preferentially via a central line or AV fistula.

▪ Monoclonal Antibodies (OKT3)

Monoclonal anti–T-cell antibodies produced from murine hybridomas to the T3 antigen of T lymphocytes have been successfully used for the treatment of acute rejection episodes. Again, anaphylactoid reactions can occur, and most patients will develop antimouse antibodies, making it useful for only one course of treatment.

Perioperative Considerations

The usual preoperative laboratory tests, including a urine culture, chest radiograph, and electrocardiogram (ECG), should be obtained. Most patients will require preoperative dialysis. Immunosuppressive medications should be started preoperatively as dictated by the prescribed protocol. Prophylactic antibiotics should be given on call to the operating room. A living related donor should be kept well hydrated with optimal urine output. An 18 F Foley catheter is placed in the recipient after induction of anesthesia. Crystalloids without potassium should be given to the recipient conservatively; however, a systolic blood pressure above 120 mm Hg should be maintained during revascularization.

Complications

Early oligoanuria after renal transplantation requires immediate evaluation.

1. Check Foley catheter for obstruction—hand irrigate.
2. Check for signs of dehydration and central venous pressure. Give fluid challenge if suggestive (500 mL normal saline over a 1-hour period).
3. Check output of surgical drains for possible urine leak.
4. Perform MAG3 or DTPA renal scan to evaluate renal perfusion.
5. Perform Doppler ultrasound of graft to rule out obstructive uropathy, to assess blood flow to the graft, and to evaluate for signs of rejection (e.g., enlargement from edema, indistinct corticomedullary junction, and loss of central renal-sinus fat echo).
6. Perform renal biopsy when poor function persists or diagnosis remains in doubt.

▦ Acute Tubular Necrosis

ATN is the most common cause of early oliguria or anuria after transplantation and is the result of ischemic insult to the kidney. Recovery will generally occur within 3 to 6 weeks; however, a renal biopsy may be helpful to rule out rejection. The diagnosis is made primarily by exclusion.

▦ Cyclosporine or Tacrolimus Nephrotoxicity

Cyclosporine or tacrolimus nephrotoxicity produces a difficult diagnostic dilemma in evaluating poor function in the postoperative period. Differentiating among ATN, acute rejection, and drug-induced nephrotoxicity is not easy. It has no pathognomonic features and does not correlate with drug blood levels. Diagnosis is usually made by a process of exclusion, often necessitating renal biopsy. Patients are managed by switching to azathioprine.

▦ Rejection

Hyperacute or Accelerated Rejection.

Hyperacute rejection is generally an irreversible process that begins within minutes to hours after transplantation and is the result of presensitization of the recipient with cytotoxic antibodies to donor ABO or HLA antigens.

Acute Rejection

Acute rejection occurs within 3 months after transplantation and is clinically characterized by fever, swelling, and tenderness over the graft, with decreased function and urine output. Hypertension also may be present.

Management of Acute Rejection

1. Steroid pulses—methylprednisolone (Solu-Medrol) 1 g IV qd × 3 days
2. ATG— antithymocyte globulin (Thymoglobulin)
3. OKT3—monoclonal anti–T-cell antibodies

Chronic Rejection

Chronic rejection results in a gradual deterioration of function, months to years after transplantation, without clear evidence of a rejection episode.

■ Surgical Complications

Vascular Complications

Vascular complications occur infrequently after transplantation; however, when they occur, they can be disastrous and must be recognized immediately.

1. Arterial occlusion can occur within the first few postoperative days. A DTPA renal scan can help make the diagnosis. Nephrectomy is usually necessary; salvage is rare.
2. Acute hemorrhage occurring within the first few hours after transplantation can be from dehiscence of a vascular suture line or from undetected or poorly ligated vessels. Late hemorrhage is most often from a pseudoaneurysm or a mycotic aneurysm. Transplant nephrectomy is usually necessary.
3. Transplant artery stenosis may produce uncontrollable hypertension months to years after transplantation. Surgical correction is often possible.

Thrombophlebitis

Thrombophlebitis is a relatively uncommon occurrence; however, if it is suspected, ultrasound or phlebography should be performed.

Graft Rupture

Graft rupture usually occurs as spontaneous severe pain and shock from massive life-threatening hemorrhage. It is believed to be caused by acute rejection and ischemia. Immediate nephrectomy is indicated.

Lymphatic

Lymphatic drainage from the area of dissection may occasionally be excessive, resulting in leakage from the incision or surgical drains. Occasionally, more prolonged drainage can result in a lymphocele, which is best diagnosed with ultrasound. The draining fluid can be differentiated from urine by measuring its creatinine or by intravenous injection of indigo carmine, which should appear only in the urine. Most lymph drainage will spontaneously resolve; however, if a significant collection develops and compromises renal function by local compression on the graft, then percutaneous or surgical drainage should be performed.

Urologic Complications

Decreased urine output in the immediate postoperative period may be due to a blood clot in the ureter or bladder. Irrigation of the bladder should be attempted. Mechanical obstruction at the ureterovesical anastomosis is common and can be caused by edema at the anastomosis or infarction of the distal ureter. Ureteral ischemia also can result in urinary extravasation with fever and graft tenderness. Ultrasound will usually make the diagnosis. Prompt and aggressive open surgical intervention is indicated.

■ Infectious Complications

Infections are the most common and life-threatening complications for the transplant recipient. Immunosuppressive therapy coupled with leukopenia, hyperglycemia, and azotemia markedly increases the risk of serious complicated infections. Bacterial sepsis is most common; however, opportunistic infections such as those with cytomegalovirus (CMV), *Pneumocystis carinii*, or *Candida albicans* are major problems. Opportunistic infections are rare in the first posttransplant month. Treatment of infections should be aggressive with intravenous antibiotics. Cyclosporine, tacrolimus, or azathioprine should be discontinued during life-threatening infections, and corticosteroids should be given at physiologic doses.

Urinary Tract Infections

Urinary tract infections are a common source of bacterial sepsis in the posttransplant patient. Use of prophylactic antibiotics and early removal of the Foley catheter can help lessen their incidence.

Wound Infection

Wound infection must always be suspected in the posttransplant patient with high fever. The incision will often look benign, even in the face of a grossly purulent abscess. Do not underestimate the masking effect of immunosuppressive agents.

Pulmonary Infection

Pulmonary infection with gram-negative bacteria, fungi, *P. carinii*, and CMV usually appears with fever and pulmonary infiltrates.

However, CMV and *Pneumocystis* can often cause severe respiratory failure before radiographic evidence of pneumonia.

Meningitis

Meningitis will often be masked by immunosuppressive therapy. Patients with unexplained fever, dull headache, photophobia, or mental-status changes should undergo lumbar puncture. Look for *Listeria*, *Candida*, *Cryptococcus*, and *Aspergillus*.

Renovascular Hypertension

In approximately 5% to 10% of patients with hypertension, the disorder has a curable etiology, of which renovascular disease is the most common. It is important to identify this small group because these are often the most difficult hypertensive patients to manage medically and because their renal lesions are usually progressive and can lead to significant renal damage.

MECHANISMS OF RENOVASCULAR HYPERTENSION

The preponderance of experimental data suggests that the mechanism of hypertension in renovascular disease is produced by stimulation of the renin–angiotensin system.

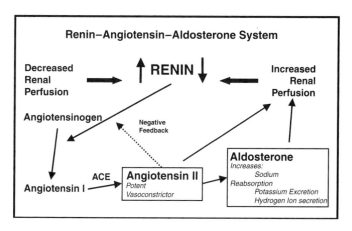

Only renal artery stenosis of a critical degree (>70%) will result in a functionally significant reduction in renal blood flow, thereby stimulating increased renin secretion. Hypertension results from the direct vasoconstrictor effect of angiotensin II and the increased vascular volume secondary to sodium retention by aldosterone.

PATHOLOGY

The major pathologic lesions producing renal artery narrowing are atherosclerosis (70%) and fibromuscular disease (30%).

Atherosclerosis

Atherosclerotic lesions cause most cases of renovascular hypertension (RVH) and usually involve the orifice and proximal 2 cm of the renal artery (i.e., near the aorta). Manifestations of generalized atherosclerosis involving the abdominal aorta and coronary, cerebral, and peripheral vasculature are usually evident.

Medial Fibroplasia

Medial fibroplasia is the second most common cause of RVH. It occurs characteristically in females aged 20 to 50 years and produces a typical multifocal "string of beads" pattern on angiography that starts in the midrenal artery and often extends into peripheral branches. Hemorrhage and dissection are rare. Correction is indicated in younger individuals.

Perimedial Fibroplasia

Perimedial fibroplasia is a progressive fibrous disease of young female patients that occurs only in the renal artery. It results in an irregular, severely stenotic lesion that often appears beaded on angiography. Surgical correction is indicated.

Intimal Fibroplasia

Intimal fibroplasia is a progressive disease that generally occurs in children or young adults, involves the proximal or middle portion of the artery, and often dissects. These lesions should be surgically corrected.

WORKUP

History

Disease onset before age 30 years and no family history of hypertension should suggest a renovascular etiology. A history of severe hypertension, headaches, or difficult medical management also is common. Patients may give a history of angina, congestive heart failure, cerebrovascular accidents, or intermittent claudication.

Factors that suggest a renovascular etiology include the following:

- Onset before age 30 years
- Sudden development or worsening of hypertension at any age
- Accelerated or malignant hypertension
- Hypertension refractory to appropriate three-drug regimen
- Extensive atherosclerotic disease
- Impaired renal function associated with hypertension or use of an angiotensin-converting enzyme inhibitor (ACEI)
- A continuous (systolic/diastolic) abdominal bruit
- A unilaterally small kidney
- Hypokalemia suggesting aldosterone hypersecretion

Physical Examination

Hypertension is defined as blood pressure of greater than 160/90 mm Hg in patients younger than 40 years and greater than 160/95 mm Hg in patients older than 40 years on three separate determinations. Check for retinopathy and abdominal or carotid bruits. Hypokalemia in the absence of diuretic therapy is highly suggestive; however, it occurs in fewer than 20% of patients.

Peripheral Plasma Renin Activity

A plasma renin activity (PRA) screening test must be performed in a highly standardized fashion because it is otherwise subject to many uncontrolled variables. Antihypertensive agents (except for β-blockers) should be discontinued at least 2 weeks before PRA screening.

▪ Screening Plasma Renin Activity

Measurement of peripheral PRA indexed to sodium excretion in a 24-hour urine sample is useful for identifying abnormally high renin secretion. The blood sample for PRA should be taken at 12 noon after 4 hours of ambulation. A low peripheral PRA is strong evidence against renal arterial disease.

▪ Captopril–Plasma Renin Activity Test (Captopril Challenge)

Captopril is an ACE inhibitor, blocking the conversion of AI to AII. In the captopril-PRA test, peripheral PRA is measured before and 1 hour after taking 25 mg captopril orally (onset of action is

10–15 minutes). Angiotensin blockade results in a marked increase in PRA and decrease in blood pressure in patients with RVH.

Rapid-Sequence Intravenous Urography

A delayed calyceal appearance time on the side with a lesion during a rapid-sequence intravenous urogram has been used to screen for patients with potential renovascular disease. However, this has been shown to have a 10% false-positive rate among patients with essential hypertension and would therefore result in incorrectly identifying an unacceptably high number of patients.

Radionuclide Renography with Angiotensin-Converting Enzyme Inhibitor

The captopril renogram has improved sensitivity and specificity over a standard renogram in identifying RVH. The patient is given 25 mg captopril PO; 1 hour later, the patient is scanned for 20 to 30 minutes after intravenous (IV) MAG3. A delay to peak activity of the scan is consistent with RVH. A repeated MAG3 scan should be performed if the ACEI renogram is abnormal.

Doppler Ultrasound

The use of Doppler ultrasound to detect renal artery stenosis has been gaining acceptance. Measurement of peak systolic velocity and the renal/aortic ratio can correctly identify high-grade renal artery stenosis. The test is technically difficult.

Renal Vein Renin Sampling

Renal vein renin (RVR) sampling is now rarely used to diagnose RVH but can be useful in localizing the more ischemic kidney in bilateral disease. RVR can demonstrate three different abnormalities.

■ Renal Vein/Renin Ratios

A renal vein/renin ratio of greater than 1.5:1 (i.e., renal vein PRA from stenotic side divided by renal vein PRA from normal side) generally predicts a correctable renal vascular lesion. This test has a false-negative rate of at least 15% and is subject to sampling error.

■ Renin Suppression

Renin is suppressed in the contralateral, noninvolved renal vein (V_{PRA}). The IVC_{PRA} can substitute for the arterial PRA (A_{PRA}).

$$V_{PRA} - IVC_{PRA} = 0$$

■ 50% Renin Increment

A renal vein PRA (V_{PRA}) increment of more than 50% on the involved side over arterial PRA (may substitute IVC_{PRA}) indicates significant RVH (assuming unilateral disease).

$$\frac{V_{PRA} - IVC_{PRA}}{IVC_{PRA}} = >0.5$$

Selective Arteriography

Selective renal arteriography is the *gold standard* for diagnosing renal artery disease. It is performed before surgical renal revascularization for a more detailed anatomic image. If percutaneous transluminal renal angioplasty is performed, angiography can be conducted at the same time.

DIAGNOSIS

Criteria for Diagnosis of Renovascular Hypertension

1. Documented sustained, fixed, diastolic hypertension
2. Demonstration of renin hypersecretion (if possible)
   a. Peripheral PRA indexed to sodium excretion or a captopril-PRA test
   b. Captopril renography
3. Demonstration of a significant vascular lesion by angiography

TREATMENT

If a curable, functional renal artery lesion is found in younger patients, surgical management is the preferred choice. Medical management is unlikely to halt progression of the disease or the potential renal damage. Vigorous medical management should be attempted in older patients with atherosclerotic RVH. Medical management of hypertension is the preferred initial treatment for a patient with medial fibroplasia. Percutaneous transluminal renal angioplasty and open surgical revascularization have both been shown to be highly successful forms of therapy. Angioplasty of the main renal artery has had excellent results in fibrous dysplasia. However, percutaneous transluminal renal angioplasty is generally unsuccessful in treating atheromatous lesions involving the ostium. Preoperative treatment of significant existing coronary or cerebrovascular occlusive disease should be considered.

It is not surprising, with the intimate anatomic and physiologic relationship between the reproductive and urinary systems, that pregnancy should have significant effects on urinary function. These changes are generally the normal consequences of pregnancy. This appreciation is helpful when called on to evaluate a urologic problem in a pregnant patient.

PHYSIOLOGIC CHANGES

Total blood volume increases during pregnancy because of a 50% increase in plasma volume and a lesser increase in red cell volume. This results in hemodilution and decreased hematocrit. With the increased blood volume, cardiac output increases early in pregnancy by 1 to 2 L/minute and is maintained until delivery. Despite the increased blood volume and cardiac output, systolic blood pressure remains essentially unchanged. This is probably due in part to the increased blood flow to the uterus (80% to the choriodecidua) and lowered peripheral vascular resistance.

During pregnancy, the mother's serum creatinine generally decreases because of a 30% to 50% increase in both renal blood flow and glomerular filtration rate (GFR). Mean serum creatinine levels of 0.46 are common. Retention of sodium and water and renal wasting of glucose and amino acids also are noted during pregnancy. These changes are generally maintained up to term. By approximately 8 postpartum weeks, most physiologic changes of pregnancy can be expected to have returned to normal.

UROLOGIC CHANGES

Pyeloureteral dilatation occurs commonly during pregnancy and is most prominent by weeks 22 to 24. The muscle-relaxing effects of increased progesterone during pregnancy is thought to play a major role in addition to mechanical factors related to the fetus. A preponderance of right-sided involvement (~75%) has been noted. Mechanical compression at the pelvic brim by the gravid uterus is the major cause. The left ureter appears to be somewhat protected from this compression by the sigmoid colon. Significant resolution of the condition can be expected within 24 to 48 hours after delivery. Urinary stasis is the most common adverse consequence of this partial obstruction; however, spontaneous rupture of the kidney has been known to occur. The bladder tends to be displaced anteriorly and superiorly by the growing uterus, producing more of an abdominal than pelvic location during pregnancy.

UROLOGIC COMPLICATIONS

Infections

▦ Asymptomatic Bacteriuria

Asymptomatic bacteriuria occurs in 2% to 7% of pregnancies. *Escherichia coli* is the infecting organism in more than 80% of cases. Complications of these asymptomatic infections include pyelonephritis, prematurity, low birth weight, anemia, hypertension, and preeclampsia. Treatment of asymptomatic bacteriuria with a 10- to 14-day course of antimicrobials has been shown to decrease the risk of developing complications. Ampicillin or cephalosporins are generally safe and effective during any phase of pregnancy. Patients with persistent bacteriuria should be treated with suppressive therapy for the remainder of the pregnancy.

▦ Symptomatic Urinary Tract Infections

Symptomatic urinary tract infections can result in significant maternal morbidity. Upper-tract obstruction and stasis are not uncommon during pregnancy and are believed to be an important predisposing factor. Pyelonephritis is a common complication of pregnancy, generally during the last two trimesters. Pyuria alone is not considered a reliable indicator of the presence or absence of infection during pregnancy. Cultures must be obtained. Treatment should be aggressive. Bacterial surveillance with frequent cultures or prolonged urinary suppression for the remainder of the pregnancy should be conducted because of the high incidence of recurrent infections.

▦ Vaginitis

The high levels of estrogens that are present during pregnancy are associated with increased vulvovaginal candidiasis. *Trichomonas* vaginitis during pregnancy should be treated with clotrimazole vaginal suppositories. Metronidazole has been demonstrated to be carcinogenic in animal studies, and it diffuses readily across the placenta.

■ Sexually Transmitted Disease

Chlamydial infection can cause cervicitis and pelvic inflammatory disease (PID). Fetal conjunctivitis is a common sequela if left untreated. Erythromycin is the drug of choice during pregnancy because of less fetal toxicity. Gonorrhea also is common in pregnancy. Diagnosis is made by smear and culture of cervical and urethral discharge. Treatment is aqueous procaine penicillin G, 4.8 million units intramuscularly, with oral probenecid.

■ Antibiotic Choices

All antibiotics cross the placental barrier to various degrees. Penicillin derivatives and cephalosporins have been shown to have minimal toxic effects to both mother and fetus and are therefore commonly used. Nitrofurantoins also are highly effective for simple urinary tract infections of pregnancy but can cause nausea and vomiting. Aminoglycosides can be used for pyelonephritis in pregnancy when other less toxic choices are unsuitable. However, because of their potential side effects of nephrotoxicity and ototoxicity, they must be used with caution in patients with renal insufficiency. Tetracyclines have numerous side effects, such as teratogenic potential and staining of the teeth, and should be avoided. Trimethoprim-sulfamethoxazole combinations are effective but should be avoided near term.

Stones

Pregnant patients who present with renal colic and microscopic hematuria should undergo renal ultrasound. If hydronephrosis is present, presumption of a ureteral calculus can be made. Fifty percent of these stones can be expected to pass spontaneously. If renal colic fails to resolve with hydration and analgesics or in the setting of severe obstruction or sepsis, then retrograde placement of a silicone double-J ureteral stent under local anesthesia may be attempted. Retrograde internal stent passage may be difficult during the third trimester, making a percutaneous approach advantageous. Radiographic studies may be necessary. A plain abdominal film [kidney, ureter, and bladder (KUB)] exposes the fetus to only 200 mrad. A limited excretory urogram, consisting of one plain film and a 30-minute film to determine obstruction, is sometimes warranted. A nuclear renogram is an alternative to intravenous urogram. It limits maternal and fetal radiation exposure at the expense of anatomic definition.

Complications of Cesarean Section

Unrecognized injury to the urinary tract can occur during a cesarean section. The bladder is most commonly involved, resulting in a vesicovaginal fistula. These patients will present with urinary incontinence after surgery. If the injury is recognized within 2 to 3 days of surgery, repair should be attempted promptly; otherwise, definitive treatment should be delayed for 2 to 3 months. Ureteral injury, more commonly on the left, can result in a fistulous communication between the ureter and the vagina or uterine corpus. Alternatively, the ureter may be inadvertently ligated in the course of controlling bleeding.

PREGNANCY IN TRANSPLANTATION

Pregnancy in the transplant recipient is a high-risk situation with increased perinatal morbidity and maternal complications, including graft rejection. Fetal complications also are high, with as many as 50% of these infants being born prematurely. However, because many successful pregnancies have been reported in transplant recipients, most centers will cautiously sanction pregnancy in selected patients with good physical and psychological health and who are at least 2 years after transplant.

Interstitial Cystitis

Interstitial cystitis (IC) is probably the least understood and most controversial of all urologic diseases. Even an agreed-on definition of the syndrome is not accepted; however, it is universally accepted that *IC is a diagnosis of exclusion*. The most commonly recognized symptoms are urgency, frequency, and suprapubic pain on bladder filling in the absence of any other reasonable causation. Hematuria has been reported in 20% to 30% of cases. It is an uncommon disease, primarily of women aged 30 to 70 years, with a 10:1 female-to-male preponderance. The etiology of IC remains obscure.

DIAGNOSIS

The diagnosis of IC is one of exclusion based entirely on clinical and cystoscopic criteria.

1. Chronic history of unexplained bladder irritability and suprapubic pain.
2. Frequency and nocturia without incontinence.
3. Negative physical examination.
4. Negative urinalysis and culture.
5. Cystoscopic findings are not mandatory:
   a. Characteristic diffuse submucosal pinpoint petechial hemorrhages (glomerulations) on cystoscopy after repeated bladder distention under 80- to 100-cm H_2O pressure (anesthesia required).
   b. Ulcerations, once thought to be common, are actually rarely found (Hunner's ulcer occurs in <5%).
6. No evidence of carcinoma in situ is found on bladder biopsy and urine cytology; interstitial mast cell infiltration, however, is frequently noted on histology.
7. Cystometric studies are essentially normal except for a small bladder capacity.

Workup

Workup should include urinalysis, urine culture, a careful voiding record, cystoscopy under anesthesia, bladder cytology or biopsy or both, intravenous urogram, and urodynamic studies. Carcinoma in situ and infection must be ruled out. Trial management with antimicrobials, anticholinergics, and antispasmodics is recommended. Relief of symptoms would exclude the diagnosis of IC.

MANAGEMENT

This disease rarely progresses and presents little threat to the patient's health. However, it can cause intolerable morbidity, at times making the patient's life unbearable. The uncertain etiology and diagnosis only worsen matters for these unfortunate patients when they are dealing with physicians. The goal of management is symptomatic relief. Both patient and physician must understand that no sure cure for IC exists. Patient education is important. Therapeutic options include the following:

1. Hydraulic distention of the bladder under anesthesia has therapeutic value in approximately 30% of patients, in addition to its diagnostic value.

2. Intravesical instillation of dimethyl sulfoxide (DMSO) is the most commonly used treatment for IC and can be expected to give at least temporary relief to 50% to 70% of patients. Fifty milliliters of a 50% solution of DMSO (Rimso-50) is instilled into the bladder by a urethral catheter and allowed to remain for 15 minutes before asking the patient to void. Instillations are repeated every 2 to 4 weeks until relief is obtained.

3. Intravesical heparin has antiinflammatory effects and inhibits angiogenesis. Dosage is 10,000 units administered intravesically in sterile water or concomitantly with DMSO.

4. The tricyclic antidepressant amitriptyline (Elavil) 12.5 to 150 mg PO daily has been beneficial for patients for whom intravesical therapy has failed.

5. Sodium pentosanpolysulfate (Elmiron) is a synthetic sulfated polysaccharide heparin analogue in oral formulation used to repair the glycosaminoglycan (GAG) layer of the bladder. Success with oral Elmiron is unpredictable. Dosage is 100 mg PO tid.

6. Transcutaneous electrical nerve stimulation (TENS) is used to relieve pain.

7. Antiinflammatory medications, such as corticosteroids and azathioprine, produce unpredictable results, and the risk of immunosuppressive complications is considered too high for routine use.

8. Augmentation cystoplasty with supratrigonal cystectomy or substitution cystoplasty is sometimes necessary as a last resort for patients with intolerable pain or small contracted bladders.

9. Dietary restrictions are unsupported by the literature; however, if patients find that their symptoms are exacerbated by specific foods or beverages, then they should be avoided.

34 Anomalies of the Genitourinary Tract

KIDNEY ANOMALIES

Agenesis

Absence of renal tissue is probably related to an interruption or loss of ureteral bud development that prevents maturation of the metanephric blastema. The major renal vessels are always absent.

■ Unilateral

Incidence is 1 in 1,100, with a slight increased frequency on the left side and an autosomal dominant inheritance noted in recent studies. Absence of the ipsilateral hemitrigone is usually diagnostic; however, a normal trigone does not rule out renal agenesis. The diagnosis is made with renal scan and ultrasound. A high association with other congenital anomalies, such as absence of vas deferens in male patients and absence or hypoplasia of the tubes, ovaries, uterus, or vagina (Meyer-Rokitansky syndrome) in female patients on the affected side, is noted. Gastrointestinal anomalies, such as imperforate anus, also are found.

■ Bilateral

This rare condition is incompatible with life.

■ Potter's Syndrome

Absence of intrauterine urine production results in oligohydramnios; death is usually secondary to pulmonary hypoplasia. Characteristic Potter's facies is noted.

Anomalies of Rotation

Malrotation generally occurs around the vertical axis, with persistent anterior position of the renal pelvis being the most common type. It may be unilateral or bilateral and is often associated with ectopy or fusion. Bizarre urograms result.

Anomalies of Position and Fusion

Renal ectopy can be classified as simple (kidney on its normal side) or crossed ectopy (on the contralateral side) with or without fusion. Fusion is defined as the anatomic union of two or more kidneys.

▇ Pelvic Kidneys

Pelvic kidney is the most recognizable ectopic kidney, with an incidence of 1 in 2,000, and usually occurs in male patients on the left side. Fifty percent of these will be pathologic with poor function, and 10% are solitary. Other coincident genitourinary anomalies, such as cryptorchidism or absence of the vagina, are common. These kidneys are difficult to identify on intravenous urogram (IVU) because of their poor function and position against the bony pelvis. Reflux is common. A voiding cystourethrogram (VCUG) can help make the diagnosis.

▇ Thoracic Kidneys

Thoracic kidneys are extremely rare; most occur in male patients on the left side.

▇ Crossed Renal Ectopia

These kidneys are more commonly fused than not fused and are usually on the right, with the crossed kidney lying inferiorly. A 2:1 male preponderance is noted. The ureteral orifices are located normally. The shape of the fused kidney can be quite unusual.

▇ Horseshoe Kidney

Horseshoe kidney is the most common type of fusion, occurring in 1 in 400, with 90% fused at the lower poles. They are often associated with other urogenital anomalies and an increased incidence of renal pelvic tumors. One third of patients remain asymptomatic, whereas others may present with symptoms of hydronephrosis [ureteropelvic junction (UPJ) obstruction], infection, or stones. The renal axis is shifted on kidney, ureter, and bladder (KUB) film so that the lower poles are closer to the vertebral bodies. The ureters lie anterior to the renal pelvis and isthmus on IVU. Reflux and UPJ obstruction occur often. Ureteroneocystostomy to treat reflux may be necessary. Dividing the renal isthmus is usually not necessary.

Renal Hypoplasia

Hypoplasia refers to reduced renal mass (i.e., fewer than normal cells or nephrons) without histologic evidence of dysplasia.

■ Oligomeganephronia

Oligomeganephronia is a congenital renal disease occurring primarily in male infants (3:1), with progressive renal failure by age 12 to 15 years. The kidneys have fewer than normal nephrons (oligonephronia) but are hypertrophied (mega). Patients are treated medically with high fluid intake and correction of salt loss until eventually dialysis and transplantation are required.

Renal Dysplasia

Dysplasia is a form of abnormal renal morphogenesis characterized histologically by primitive ducts and cartilage. Varying degrees of hypoplasia are always present. Most hypodysplastic kidneys have ectopic ureteral orifices. The more ectopic the orifice, the greater the degree of dysplasia.

Renal Cystic Diseases

Many different classification schemes have been advanced. The major entities follow.

■ Autosomal Recessive Polycystic Kidney Disease

Autosomal recessive (infantile) polycystic kidney disease (ARPKD) is a rare anomaly with no sex predilection. Neither parent shows evidence of the disease, and siblings of either sex have a 1 in 4 chance of being affected. Ultrasound will show massively enlarged kidneys bilaterally, and IVU will show characteristic radial or medullary streaking of the nephrogram from cystic dilatation of the collecting tubules. Renal insufficiency occurs early. Infants with evidence of the disease at birth often die within the first 2 months. Patients will have some form of liver disease, ranging from periportal biliary ectasia to congenital hepatic fibrosis. A liver biopsy can establish the diagnosis. For those patients who survive infancy (50%), the course and progression of the disease are variable; however, cardiac, renal, and hepatic failure can be expected. ARPKD has no known cure.

■ Autosomal Dominant Polycystic Kidney Disease

Autosomal dominant (adult) polycystic kidney disease (ADPKD) is the most common form of cystic kidney disease in humans and is responsible for approximately 10% of all cases of end-stage renal disease (ESRD). Approximately 500,000 Americans have been diagnosed. The trait has 100% penetrance, and 50% of an affected individual's offspring also will be affected. This condition is characterized by diffuse bilateral progressive cystic degeneration of the kidneys, hypertension, and progressive renal failure. Most cases are identified between the ages of 30 and 50 years. Typical signs or symptoms include gross or microscopic hematuria, flank pain, gastrointestinal symptoms (colonic diverticula), renal colic (from clots or stones), and hypertension. Associated anomalies include hepatic cysts or fibrosis, berry aneurysms (10% to 40%), mitral valve prolapse, and colonic diverticulosis.

Treatment

Hypertension should be managed aggressively. Stones develop in 20% to 30% of patients with ADPKD and should be treated conservatively with urine alkalinization and extracorporeal shock wave lithotripsy (ESWL). Unnecessary instrumentation of the urinary tract should be avoided because of the high risk of infection in polycystic kidneys. Upper-tract infection is more successfully managed with lipid soluble antibiotics such as trimethoprim–sulfamethoxazole (TMP-SMX) or fluoroquinolones. Renewed interest in surgical/laparoscopic cyst unroofing has been beneficial in relieving pain associated with the cysts. Renal failure can be managed with dialysis or renal transplantation.

▓ Congenital Multicystic Kidney Disease

Congenital multicystic kidney disease is a common benign dysplastic malformation of the fetal kidney secondary to obstruction from ureteropelvic occlusion, ureteral atresia, or agenesis. It presents predominantly in male infants, on the left side, with a large, unilateral, multicystic, nonfunctioning renal abdominal mass. A 10% to 15% incidence of significant anomalies of the contralateral upper urinary tract is found. Elective surgical excision is indicated if the mass interferes with respiration or alimentation of the child or is associated with significant hypertension. Otherwise, attention is directed primarily toward identifying any abnormalities of the contralateral urinary tract.

▓ Simple Cysts (Retention Cysts)

The most common cystic lesions of the kidney, simple cysts, may be solitary or multiple, unilateral or bilateral. They present clinically as an abdominal mass or more commonly as an incidental finding on ultrasound, IVU, or computed tomography (CT) scan. Differentiation among cystic neoplasms, lymphatic cysts, perirenal effusions, and renal abscesses must be made, in addition to polycystic disease, when they are multiple. A cystic renal cell carcinoma must be ruled out.

A simple cyst is characteristically unilocular, avascular, smooth walled, and filled with a clear fluid with low fat and protein content and a low lactic dehydrogenase with no malignant cells on cytology. Most complex cysts (Bosniak III or IV) on ultrasound or CT should undergo surgical exploration (see Chapter 15).

■ Medullary Sponge Kidney

Medullary sponge kidney is a congenital deformity of the renal medulla consisting of multiple, puddle-like dilatations of the collecting ducts in the papillae on IVU. These ectatic tubules are not true cysts but give a characteristic fan-shaped pyramidal blush on IVU that is diagnostic. The disease is bilateral in 75% of patients. Although its course and progression are generally benign, its clinical importance is its predisposition to calcium phosphate nephrolithiasis in the adult, presenting with renal colic and hematuria secondary to stone passage. Treatment consists of preventing infection and stone formation.

■ Tuberous Sclerosis (Bourneville's Disease)

Tuberous sclerosis is a familial autosomal dominant condition characterized by congenital tumors. Clinical features include the following:
- Facial nevi ("sebaceous adenoma")
- Recurrent convulsive seizures
- Mental retardation
- Multiple angiomyolipomas in up to 50%
- Occasionally, diffuse renal cystic disease that can result in chronic renal failure.

■ von Hippel–Lindau Disease

von Hippel–Lindau disease is an autosomal dominantly inherited syndrome manifested by retinal and cerebellar hemangioblastomas; cysts of the kidney, pancreas, and epididymis; pheochromocytomas; and renal cell carcinoma in 30% to 40% of patients. Renal cysts are often multiple and bilateral and appear to be precursors of malignant tumors. Yearly abdominal CT is recommended in these patients because of the high incidence of renal cell carcinomas. Shelling out these tumors rather than radical surgery is appropriate in view of their multiplicity.

■ Acquired Renal Cystic Disease

Acquired renal cystic disease is the appearance of bilateral multiple cysts in previously noncystic native kidneys of patients with ESRD. The risk of developing these cysts appears to be related to uremic toxins. Their significance lies in their apparent premalignant nature. The incidence of renal cell carcinoma is three to six times greater in patients on dialysis. Complaints of flank pain or hematuria or both in an ESRD patient should be investigated for acquired renal cystic disease or renal cell carcinoma.

Anomalies of the Collecting System

■ Extrarenal Pelvis

Extrarenal pelvis predisposes to stasis, infection, and stone formation.

■ Bifid Pelvis

Bifid pelvis is a normal variant that occurs in 10% of the population.

■ Congenital Calyceal Diverticulum

Congenital calyceal diverticulum is a cystic cavity lying in the peripheral renal parenchyma connected to a calyx or the renal pelvis. Distention with urine can cause pain; however, infection and stone formation secondary to stasis are the most common complications. Diagnosis is made with IVU, retrograde pyelogram, or CT scan.

■ Hydrocalycosis

Hydrocalycosis is a rare cystic dilatation of a major calyx secondary to obstruction at the level of the infundibulum.

■ Congenital Megacalyces

Congenital megacalyces is a stable malformation of markedly enlarged calyceal cavities without evidence of obstruction. It occurs in male patients, in a 6:1 ratio, is highly associated with megaureter, and predisposes to infection and stones. The diagnosis is made with IVU, with a negative furosemide (Lasix) renal scan or Whitaker test. Preventing infection and stone formation with a high fluid intake is the goal of management.

URETERAL ANOMALIES

Ureteropelvic Junction Obstruction

Obstruction at the UPJ is a common congenital anomaly resulting in an obstruction to urine flow of varying degrees. Lesser degrees of obstruction become symptomatic only with diuresis. UPJ obstruction occurs more commonly in male patients (2:1), with most cases diagnosed within the first year of life. Left-sided lesions predominate, and up to 40% are bilateral. Few cases are noted after puberty and into adulthood.

■ Etiologies

1. Intrinsic lesion of the circular smooth muscle of the UPJ
2. Extrinsic compression by an aberrant, accessory, or early-branching vessel to the lower pole
3. Obstruction secondary to severe reflux, resulting in kinking of a tortuous ureter

■ Diagnosis

Today UPJ obstruction is diagnosed almost exclusively in the prenatal period because of the wide use of maternal ultrasonography. Renal ultrasound should be repeated postnatally after the first few weeks of life. Infants may present with an asymptomatic abdominal mass or urosepsis. Adults may have episodic flank pain, especially during diuresis. Doppler ultrasound measurement of the vascular resistive index (>0.70) can help identify significant obstruction in infants. An IVU will show a markedly hydronephrotic kidney with abrupt cutoff at the UPJ. A diuretic MAG3 or diethylenetriaminepentaacetate (DTPA) renogram is often helpful in equivocal cases. A VCUG is mandatory to rule out severe reflux as the cause of hydronephrosis. A dimethylsulfoxide (DMSA) renal scan may sometimes be helpful to determine the degree of renal function in the obstructed kidney. A Whitaker test can be used on occasion if a nephrostomy tube is in place.

■ Treatment

Pyeloplasty is the recommended treatment by open or laparoscopic approaches. Early versus late pyeloplasty is controversial in very young patients. A nephrectomy may be indicated if less than 10% renal function remains.

Ureteral Duplication

Ureteral duplication is the most frequent anomaly of the urinary tract and is twice as common in female as in male patients. The ureteral orifice of the upper renal segment drains inferiorly and medially to the orifice of the lower segment (Meyer-Weigert law). The orifice draining the upper segment is often obstructed, whereas the orifice of the lower segment generally refluxes. Duplication is usually discovered on an IVU.

Ectopic Ureter

An ectopic ureter is one that opens in some location other than the bladder.
- 80% are associated with a duplicated system, usually in female patients.
- 20% are single ectopic ureters usually occurring in male patients with an absent hemitrigone.
- Most common sites for insertion of the ectopic orifice in female patients are the urethra, vestibule, and vagina, and present as urinary incontinence.
- Most common sites for insertion of the ectopic orifice in male patients are the posterior urethra and seminal vesicles, often remaining unrecognized until late in life.

Continuous incontinence in an otherwise normal female patient should suggest an ectopic ureteral orifice. Male patients present with urinary tract infections, not incontinence.

▦ Diagnosis

An IVU with tomography and delayed films, VCUG, ultrasound, and cystourethroscopy should be obtained. Intravenous indigo carmine during urethroscopy can help locate the ectopic orifice. A DMSA renal scan may be helpful in differentiating function between the upper and lower poles. Approximately 10% to 20% of ectopic orifices will not be found without surgical exploration.

▦ Treatment

Treatment is either partial nephroureterectomy of the nonfunctioning upper-pole component or pyelopyelostomy with only a distal ureterectomy if the upper pole functions. A nephrectomy may be necessary in a single system.

Ureterocele

A ureterocele is a congenital cystic ballooning of the terminal submucosal ureter. It is classified as simple or ectopic.

▦ Simple (Orthotopic) Ureteroceles

This type represents about 30% of all ureteroceles and occurs primarily in adult men. The ureter is normally placed in the trigone. Patients present with infection, and reflux is uncommon.

▓ Ectopic Ureterocele

Ectopic ureterocele represents about 70% of all ureteroceles, occurring mainly in girls, with a left predominance; 10% are bilateral. It arises from the dysplastic upper-pole ectopic ureter of a duplicated system with little or no function. The orifice is often at the bladder neck or within the urethra. It can obstruct the ipsilateral lower pole or contralateral ureter and occasionally the bladder neck. This is a serious anomaly, with children often seen in the first few months of life with infection.

Diagnosis

Ureteroceles are increasingly being discovered on prenatal ultrasound. Ureteroceles are easily visualized on the cystogram phase of an IVU. The classic nonopaque filling defect of the cobra-head or spring-onion deformity can be confused with a tumor, stone, blood clot, or gas in the rectum. A VCUG can assess for reflux (40%). Diagnosis is confirmed by cystoscopy. A renal scan should be performed to evaluate renal function.

Treatment

Treatment must be tailored to the patient's altered anatomy and physiology.

Simple ureteroceles can be approached intravesically, with excision and reimplantation of the distal ureter. Ectopic ureteroceles are approached like ectopic ureters. If upper-pole function is poor, an upper-pole partial nephrectomy is performed with partial or complete ureterectomy. Eventual reimplantation of the lower-pole ureter may be necessary if reflux is severe or persistent. A complete nephroureterectomy may be necessary if the entire kidney is nonfunctional.

Retrocaval Ureter

A retrocaval or circumcaval ureter is an uncommon congenital anomaly whereby the right ureter deviates medially behind the inferior vena cava, encircling the cava and passing in front of it, before resuming its normal lateral course to the bladder. Patients present with evidence of obstruction in the third or fourth decade of life.

▓ Diagnosis

An IVU generally will not show the retrocaval part of the ureter. A retrograde ureterogram will typically demonstrate an S-shaped ureter coursing toward the cava at the point of obstruction.

■ Treatment

Surgical management entails ureteral division with ureteroureteral anastomosis.

Megaureter

Megaureter or "big" ureter is a term that most urologists use to refer to primary ureteral dilatation in the absence of extraureteral disease. However, the term has been extended to include the classification of all major ureterectasis with emphasis on differentiating obstructed from nonobstructed varieties. Most children with megaureter will present with urinary tract infection, hematuria, or a flank mass; 25% of cases are bilateral.

■ Classification

The international classification of megaureter includes three major categories:

- Obstructed megaureter can be from primary intrinsic ureteral obstruction, usually by an extravesical adynamic ureteral segment, or secondary to urethral obstruction as with valves, prolapsing ureterocele, calculi, granulomatous disease, or other extrinsic causes;
- Refluxing megaureter is from either primary intrinsic ureteral reflux or reflux secondary to bladder-outlet obstruction or neurogenic bladder;
- Nonrefluxing, nonobstructed megaureter is a congenital idiopathic ureteral dilatation often associated with megacalycosis.

■ Workup

Workup usually begins with an ultrasound and VCUG to determine the degree of ureterectasis and the presence or absence of reflux. Obstruction can be determined by a furosemide (Lasix) renal scan or IVU or a Whitaker test in the event of an equivocal scan.

■ Treatment

Most patients with primary megaureter have the nonrefluxing, nonobstructing type that needs no surgical intervention. These patients should be followed up, with surgery reserved for those with evidence of progressive renal parenchymal damage or recurrent infections. Primary obstructive megaureter requires surgical correction, commonly by tapering the lowermost 5 cm of ureter with reimplantation. Any and all extraureteral causes of obstruction should also be relieved. Refluxing megaureter can be managed with either medical surveillance or operative correction (see Chapter 35).

URACHUS

The urachus is a tubular structure extending from the anterior bladder wall to the umbilicus. It lies on the anterior abdominal wall between the two umbilical arteries in the space of Retzius between the peritoneum and transversalis fascia. It normally involutes into a solid cord by the fourth or fifth month of gestation.

Patent Urachus

A patent urachus is a rare congenital anomaly in which the urachus fails to involute, resulting in an open communication between the bladder and the umbilicus. It presents in the neonatal period with constant or intermittent leakage of urine from the umbilicus. The diagnosis can be confirmed by measuring creatinine of the discharge fluid, VCUG, fistulogram, or by instilling colored dye into the bladder. Spontaneous closure may occur if leakage is small; otherwise, complete excision of the tract is usually required.

Urachal Cyst

A urachal cyst develops in a partially obliterated urachus, usually in the lower third. It presents commonly in adult life with suprapubic pain, tenderness, fever, voiding symptoms, and a palpable mass. The diagnosis is made with ultrasound, IVU, CT, and VCUG. Treatment consists of incision and drainage or marsupialization with delayed excision.

Umbilical Sinus

An umbilical sinus is a chronically infected urachal cyst that drains to the umbilicus. The diagnosis is made by sinogram and cystogram. Treatment consists of antibiotics and excision of the sinus tract.

BLADDER AND URETHRAL ANOMALIES

Exstrophy Complex

Exstrophy is a rare congenital defect resulting in a spectrum of anomalies of the urogenital and musculoskeletal system secondary to persistence of the cloacal membrane in utero. It occurs in approximately 1 in 30,000 live births, with a male predominance of 3:1. Three major subgroups represent different degrees of severity of the defect.

▪ Cloacal Exstrophy (10%)

Cloacal exstrophy is the most severe and distressing of these defects, involving a massive defect of the anterior abdominal wall with exposed bladder, ileocecal bowel, and a short blind-ending colonic segment with imperforate anus. Myelomeningoceles are present in 50%. Management of these patients' severe problems has recently become more aggressive, with encouraging successes.

▪ Classic Bladder Exstrophy (60%)

Classic bladder exstrophy presents as a protruding red mass in the suprapubic region, which is the exposed back wall and trigone of the bladder, and an epispadiac urethra leaking urine. Associated defects include a widely separated pubic symphysis and lower rectus muscles, frequent bilateral indirect inguinal hernias and retractile testes, and rectal prolapse in 15% to 20%. Upper tracts are generally normal.

Treatment

The prognosis for patients with classic bladder exstrophy is excellent, with normal life expectancies and good quality of life. All patients deserve an attempt at staged functional reconstruction, preferably in the first 48 hours of life to minimize bladder damage secondary to environmental exposure, and may avoid the need for iliac osteotomies. The most important part of their treatment is to refer them to a pediatric urologist who has experience with exstrophy immediately after birth.

▪ Epispadias (30%)

Epispadias is the least severe defect with only an open urethra on the dorsum of the penis and a lesser degree of separation of the pubic symphysis. Approximately 90% will have vesicoureteral reflux, and 75% will present with incontinence.

Urethral Valves

▪ Posterior Urethral Valves

Posterior urethral valves are the most common etiology of bladder-outlet obstruction in boys. They are congenital membrane-like structures located in the distal prostatic urethra covered by transitional epithelium. They present with varying degrees of obstruction and are usually diagnosed within the first year of life. Infants with severe degrees of obstruction can present with a palpable bladder and bilateral hydronephrotic flank masses, urinary ascites, renal insufficiency, and infection.

Classification

Classification by H. H. Young, in 1919, into three types is still used.

- Type I valves are most common (95%). They appear as mucosal sails extending from either side of the distal verumontanum and attaching to the anterolateral walls of the membranous urethra.
- Type II valves are more proximal, arising from the verumontanum and passing toward the bladder neck. They are generally not believed to be a clinically significant cause of obstruction.
- Type III valves are membrane-like structures, usually with a small central perforation, and are not attached to the verumontanum.

Diagnosis

Diagnosis is increasingly made with prenatal ultrasound. Postnatal diagnosis is often made with ultrasound or a VCUG demonstrating a dilated and elongated posterior urethra and reflux in about 50%. A renal scan is often helpful. Direct visualization can be made during cystourethroscopy, along with noting bladder trabeculation.

Management

Preservation of renal function and prevention of infection must guide management. Immediate relief of obstruction should be undertaken without delay with catheter drainage. Healthy, uninfected children can have simple endoscopic destruction of the valves. Infants with evidence of severe obstruction, complicated by infection and persistent renal insufficiency after a period of catheter drainage, can be managed by primary high urinary diversion, as with cutaneous vesicostomy or loop ureterostomies, or even bilateral nephrostomy tubes. Delayed secondary endoscopic destruction can be performed later.

■ Anterior Urethral Valves

Anterior urethral valves are far less common and generally produce less damage from obstruction. Boys will typically present with signs of bladder-outlet obstruction, infection, or a palpable ventral urethral swelling at the penoscrotal junction during or after voiding. Urethral distention proximal to the valve will result in a saccular diverticulum in the bulbar urethra. Diagnosis is made with a VCUG. The valvelike obstruction can be relieved by endoscopic electroresection; however, an associated diverticulum will generally require open excision and urethroplasty.

PENIS

Hypospadias

Hypospadias is a congenital anomaly of the penis resulting from an incomplete development of the anterior urethra. The defect involves primarily an abnormal urethral opening, proximal to its normal location and often with an associated ventral chordee or curvature of the penis. It can be expected to occur in about 1 of every 300 live male births and is believed to have a multifactorial genetic mode of inheritance.

■ Familial Incidence

- 7% will have a father with hypospadias.
- 14% will have a brother with hypospadias.
- 21% will have a second family member with hypospadias.

■ Classification

Classification is simply by anatomic description of the meatal position (glanular, coronal, distal shaft, mid-shaft, proximal shaft, penoscrotal, scrotal, and perineal) and the degree of chordee (mild, moderate, and severe). The severity of the chordee usually increases with more proximal meatal openings. About 75% of cases can be expected to be of the glanular or coronal types.

■ Associated Anomalies

Undescended testes occur in about 10% of cases; inguinal hernias also occur in about 10% of cases. In the more proximal varieties of hypospadias, undescended testes occur in up to 30% of cases. Upper-tract anomalies occur in about 5%, and other system anomalies are even less common; however, their presence should alert one to evaluate the upper urinary tract fully. Intersex must be considered in patients with severe forms of hypospadias and ambiguous genitalia or nonpalpable testes.

■ Management

More than 100 variations of procedures are described for the surgical correction of hypospadias. All must contend with functional and plastic repair of the urethra and correction of chordee (orthoplasty). The optimal time for repair is between ages 6 and 12 months. Surgical complications include urethrocutaneous fistula, persistent chordee, urethral stricture, diverticula, and meatal stenosis.

Epispadias

Epispadias is a rare congenital anomaly and the least severe form of the exstrophy complex. The malformed open urethra will lie on the dorsal surface of the penis, and diastasis of the symphysis pubis and rectus muscles commonly occurs. It affects predominantly males, 5:1. Vesicoureteral reflux is noted in 75%.

■ Classification

- Glanular epispadias (15%) is the rarest, with only a minor urethral defect on the dorsum of the glans penis.
- Penile epispadias (25%) is noted by an open distal urethra on the dorsal surface of the penis. Half can be expected to have a widened symphysis; however, continence is not a problem in these children.
- Penopubic epispadias (60%) will have the entire urethra open along the dorsal surface of the penis. The pubic symphysis is separated, and urinary incontinence is the rule. Dorsal penile chordee is common, and portions of the bladder may prolapse through the wide-open prostatic urethra. This is the most significant form of isolated epispadias noted in female patients and is referred to as subsymphyseal epispadias. The labia will not be fused, and the clitoris is bifid.

■ Management

Management is dictated by the degree of deformity. Glanular and penile epispadias will require elective urethroplasty and release of dorsal chordee. Penopubic epispadias with incontinence will require more-extensive reconstruction, similar to that for classic exstrophy, and usually includes a bladder-neck plasty, urethroplasty, and ureteral reimplants, as needed. Continence can be achieved in 60% to 80%.

CRYPTORCHIDISM

Cryptorchidism is one of the most common disorders in pediatric urology. It has been observed to occur in 3% of term infants and 30% of premature infants. By age 1 year, most of these testes will have spontaneously descended, leaving a true incidence of about 1% of the male population. Ten percent of cases are bilateral, 3%

of which will have one or both testes absent. The etiology is unclear; however, an association with low birth weight has been established. Many genetically inherited diseases have a high association with cryptorchidism, yet most cases of undescended testis are isolated with no evidence of a genetic component (see Chapter 11).

IMPERFORATE ANUS

The imperforate anus is a spectrum of congenital anomalies resulting from a failure of the normal descent of the urorectal septum in utero. The major clinical feature is the loss of a normal anal opening on the perineum, ranging between only minor anal stenosis to complete anal or rectal agenesis. Its incidence is reported at 1 in 5,000 births.

Two Major Clinical Subgroups

Two types of imperforate anus are recognized, based on the level of the blind-ending colonic pouch relative to the pelvic floor or levator ani muscles.

High or Supralevator Lesions

- High or supralevator lesions, primarily owing to rectal agenesis, have a high association with other anomalies.
- A high incidence of fistulas, usually rectourethral in male patients or rectovaginal in female patients, are noted.
- Associated urologic anomalies occur in 50%.
- A high incidence of upper-tract abnormalities (30%), including unilateral renal agenesis, hypoplasia, dysplasia, reflux, and ureteral obstruction, are found.
- Neuropathic bladders occur in 10%, secondary to congenital sacral abnormalities or from surgical dissection at rectal pull-through procedures (iatrogenic).
- Tracheoesophageal fistula or atresia is noted in approximately 10%.
- Lumbosacral spine abnormalities occur in 30% to 40%.
- Cardiac anomalies occur in 7%.

Low or Infralevator Lesions

Low or infralevator lesions, primarily owing to anal agenesis, have a much lower incidence of sacral or urologic abnormalities. Upper-tract abnormalities occur in only 10%.

Workup

Examine the perineum. Any evidence of meconium staining suggests a low lesion. Meconium in the urine suggests a high lesion. Obtain an abdominal–renal ultrasound, renal scan, and VCUG, and perform cystourethroscopy before surgery. Be suspicious for hyperchloremic acidosis, particularly with high lesions.

Treatment

High lesions are best managed by a diverting colostomy and later rectal pull-through that is delayed for 6 to 12 months. Low lesions may be treated with a primary anoplasty. If reflux is significant, suppressive antibiotics, with or without cutaneous vesicostomy, may be necessary.

PRUNE-BELLY SYNDROME

The prune-belly syndrome (also known as Eagle-Barrett syndrome) is a rare congenital anomaly with an incidence of 1 in 50,000 live births that occurs almost exclusively in male patients (only 3% in female patients).

Major Characteristics

- Abdominal-wall defect from muscular deficiency ranging from partial hypoplasia to complete absence, giving the classic wrinkled appearance with bulging flanks
- Dilated and tortuous ureters, particularly at the lower end, with accompanying reflux in most cases
- Asymmetrical renal dysplasia and hydronephrosis
- Cryptorchidism with bilateral intraabdominal testes (orchiopexy is difficult because of short spermatic vessels)
- Wide and dilated bladder neck and posterior urethra secondary to prostatic hypoplasia—urethral valves are rare; occasionally urethral atresia, usually associated with a patent urachus
- Large, thick-walled, irregularly shaped bladder, usually with a pseudodiverticulum at the dome and widely separated refluxing ureteral orifices

Associated Anomalies

- Frequent malrotation of the gastrointestinal tract and, occasionally, imperforate anus

- Cardiac abnormalities (in 10%), including ventricular septal defects, atrial septal defects, and tetralogy of Fallot
- Pulmonary complications such as pneumothorax and pulmonary hypoplasia secondary to severe renal dysplasia and oligohydramnios

Classification of Prune-Belly Syndrome

Category I—most severe form with oligohydramnios and pulmonary hypoplasia (poor prognosis; no surgical intervention)
Category II—classic features with uropathy and mild or unilateral renal dysplasia
Category III—mild external features and uropathy with stable renal function

Management

Most patients present in the neonatal period. Rarely are they a urologic emergency. Category I infants usually will not survive because of the severe pulmonary hypoplasia and renal dysplasia. Category III infants do well and need little urologic intervention. Management of category II infants focuses on their predisposition to urinary stasis and infection with potential renal deterioration.

▥ Workup

Electrolytes, blood urea nitrogen (BUN), creatinine, urine cultures, chest radiograph, abdominal ultrasound, renal scan, and IVU should be performed early. A VCUG may be indicated if early surgery is considered; however, instrumentation of the lower urinary tract should be avoided because of the increased risk of infection.

▥ Treatment

Maintain renal function and avoid infection. If urinary drainage is needed because of infection, then a cutaneous vesicostomy or cutaneous pyelostomy should be undertaken. Orchiopexy is usually attempted. Reduction cystoplasty is sometimes useful. Plastic repair of the abdominal wall improves body image. Long-term surveillance is mandatory.

MYELOMENINGOCELE

Myelodysplasia refers to a spectrum of congenital spinal anomalies caused by defects in neural tube closure. It occurs in 1 in 1,000 births in the United States. Failure of the posterior vertebral arches to fuse results in the development of a cystic meningocele, which contains dysplastic neural elements. The cord is frequently tethered to adjacent bony structures and does not recede with normal growth. Various degrees of myelomeningocele occur, from spina bifida occulta to spina bifida aperta. The resulting neurologic deficits include lower urinary tract dysfunction, with more than 90% of these patients having incontinence. Bladder and sphincter dysfunction occurs, including detrusor areflexia or hyperreflexia, with or without coordinated sphincter activity. The primary goals of management are to preserve renal function, prevent infection, and provide urinary control.

Workup

In addition to specific neurologic assessment, early evaluation of the upper tracts must be made in the neonatal period. Urinalysis, urine culture, and ultrasound should be obtained. If hydronephrosis is found (10%), a VCUG should be performed to look for vesicoureteral reflux. Urodynamic evaluation will eventually be necessary. Patients will need careful, periodic, close follow-up with urinalysis, culture, and imaging of the upper tracts with ultrasound or urography.

Management

Patients' disorders should be classified as either failure to empty or failure to store. Clean intermittent catheterization (CIC) is the most common mode of therapy for patients who fail to empty. Patients who fail to store can be managed with pharmacologic agents or surgical procedures to enlarge the bladder or increase outlet resistance (e.g., bladder neck plasty, slings, or artificial sphincters). Urinary diversion is a last resort. Antireflux procedures are also commonly needed.

35 Vesicoureteral Reflux

Vesicoureteral reflux (VUR) is the backward flow of urine from the bladder into the upper urinary tract. It is an abnormality that is associated with recurrent urinary tract infections and a particular form of renal damage known as reflux nephropathy. Because of its pathogenic role in reflux nephropathy, early recognition and eradication are essential. Primary reflux is the result of a congenital anomaly of the ureterovesical junction, whereas secondary reflux is the result of bladder-outlet obstruction and high intravesical pressures.

PATHOPHYSIOLOGY

The most distal 13 mm of the ureter in adults lies intravesically (5 mm in neonates), including an intramural segment within the muscular wall of the bladder and a submucosal segment lying just beneath the bladder mucosa. This intravesical segment acts as a passive flap-valve mechanism to prevent reflux. The ratio between the length of the submucosal segment and the diameter of the ureter (normal, 4:1 or 5:1) is believed to be an important factor for normal function of the antireflux mechanism. Active peristalsis of the ureter also acts to prevent reflux.

Factors associated with VUR include the following:
- A short submucosal tunnel
- Lateral placement of the ureteral orifice
- Abnormal configuration of ureteral orifice (e.g., stadium, horseshoe, and golf-hole orifices)
- Infection
- Severe bladder-outlet obstruction
- Young age
- Duplicated collecting systems (particularly from the more laterally placed orifice draining the lower pole)

Consequences of Reflux

Persistent VUR has been associated with renal damage, pyelonephritic scarring, and eventually impaired renal function, hypertension, and proteinuria. Reflux nephropathy refers to the radiologic changes of reflux including dilated calyces, renal parenchymal thinning, and scarring. Experimental and clinical data suggest that the combination of VUR and intrarenal reflux of *infected* urine into the collecting tubules of the nephron is necessary for renal damage to occur. In addition, the risk of renal scarring is greatest in children younger than 1 year and is uncommon after age 5 years. Early diagnosis and antibiotic treatment are important to prevent reflux nephropathy.

Megacystis–Megaureter Syndrome

The megacystis–megaureter syndrome is a condition characterized by a large-capacity, smooth, thin-walled bladder and massive vesicoureteral reflux in children. The massively dilated ureters and large-capacity bladder are a result of the constant recycling of large volumes of refluxed urine. The syndrome is not a problem of bladder-outlet obstruction or neurogenic bladder but is caused by massive primary vesicoureteral reflux. Therapy should be directed toward correction of the reflux.

INCIDENCE

The incidence of VUR in the general population is estimated to be less than 2%. However, in children investigated because of urinary tract infection, the incidence is between 30% and 50% and decreases with advancing age. Siblings of patients with reflux are at a much greater risk of also having reflux.

GRADING SYSTEM

The international grading system for reflux is based primarily on the radiographic appearance of the calyces on voiding cystourethrography (VCUG).

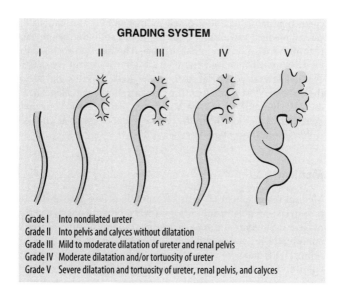

GRADING SYSTEM

| I | II | III | IV | V |

Grade I   Into nondilated ureter
Grade II   Into pelvis and calyces without dilatation
Grade III Mild to moderate dilatation of ureter and renal pelvis
Grade IV Moderate dilatation and/or tortuosity of ureter
Grade V   Severe dilatation and tortuosity of ureter, renal pelvis, and calyces

DIAGNOSIS

Urinalysis and culture should be performed early in the workup to exclude infection. The principal diagnostic test for evaluating VUR is the voiding cystourethrogram (VCUG). A nuclear cystogram is a good alternative and is more sensitive for picking up low-grade reflux; however, it does not give the anatomic detail of a VCUG and makes grading the reflux more difficult. A renal ultrasound has replaced the intravenous urography (IVU) for initial evaluation of the upper tracts in children. Dimethylsulfoxide (DMSO) renal scan is the study of choice for detecting pyelonephritis and cortical renal scarring. Cystoscopy should be performed at the time of a planned surgical repair only if indicated. Indications for cystoscopy include nonvisualization of the urethra on VCUG, uncertain ureteral location or anomaly, or localization of a paraureteral diverticulum. Urodynamic evaluation is indicated in children with secondary reflux.

MANAGEMENT

The management of patients is based on the observation that VUR has a natural tendency for spontaneous resolution. Surgical correction can often be avoided by maintaining the patient on careful medical surveillance and continuous antibiotic prophylaxis to prevent secondary renal damage. The decision for medical versus surgical management is made after a careful diagnostic evaluation, with particular focus on the grade of reflux and age of the patient. Most grade I to III refluxes resolve spontaneously, as do some in grade IV. Grade V refluxes seldom resolve on their own. Reflux is more likely to resolve spontaneously in younger children regardless of grade.

Medical

Medical management consists of continuous low-dose antibiotic prophylaxis, regular urine cultures (every 3 months), and a yearly nuclear cystogram and renal ultrasound. Medical surveillance is appropriate for young children with mild-to-moderate grades of reflux (I–III) and very young children with grade IV reflux. Ampicillin or amoxicillin is appropriate for children younger than 6 weeks, whereas trimethoprim–sulfamethoxazole can be used after 6 weeks (mature biliary system). Grade V reflux also is managed medically in newborns until the child is old enough for surgical management.

Surgical

The success rate for antireflux procedures is greater than 90% in experienced hands. Indications for early surgical intervention follow.
- Breakthrough infection despite antibiotic prophylaxis
- Poor compliance with medical regimen
- Progressive renal scarring with antibiotic prophylaxis
- A refluxing orifice within a diverticulum
- Severe reflux (grade IV or V)

Diagnostic Techniques

HISTORY AND PHYSICAL EXAMINATION

The history is the foundation of all diagnosis and should be performed in a systematic and orderly fashion to avoid errors of omission. This cannot be overemphasized. History taking should be tailored to the patient's chief complaint and should include a review of major signs and symptoms of genitourinary disease, as well as a general review of systems.

Historical Data

1. Voiding problems:
   - Storage (irritative) symptoms (frequency, urgency, nocturia)
   - Voiding (obstructive) symptoms (hesitancy; straining; dysuria; slow, weak, or intermittent stream; terminal dribbling; retention); incontinence (get details)
2. Urethral discharge (onset, color, consistency, last sexual contact)
3. Hematuria (when started, how much, how often, color)
4. Bloody ejaculation
5. Fever, chills, flank pain
6. Pyuria, pneumaturia
7. Sex-related problems
8. History of genitourinary problems—kidney, bladder, prostate, infections, stones, or difficulty urinating
9. General medical history with review of systems (cardiorespiratory, hypertension, diabetes, neurologic, gastrointestinal, and careful review of medications and allergies)

Physical Examination

Abdomen—pain or tenderness, palpable masses, auscultation for bruits, palpate for bladder
Penis—discharge, foreskin, palpable plaques, meatus

Testes—size, tenderness, palpable masses, hydrocele, spermatocele, varicocele, transillumination, beading of vas
Vaginal examination—discharges, cystocele, rectocele, enterocele, prolapse, bimanual palpation
Rectal examination—sphincter tone, prostate (size, consistency, nodules, mobility, tenderness)
Skin lesions—morphology and distribution

URINALYSIS

Urinalysis is the single most important screening test available to the urologist.

Urine Collection

Proper urine collection is necessary for accurate interpretation of urinalysis or culture. All tests must be performed on a freshly voided specimen. Urine that has been left standing becomes alkaline, with lysis of red blood cells, disintegration of casts, formation of crystals, and proliferation of bacteria.

■ Male Patients

A voided, midstream clean-catch urine sample is routine; however, split voided specimens are sometimes helpful in localizing the source of infection or hematuria (see Technique for Urine Specimen Localization, later).

■ Female Patients

A voided specimen in female patients must be obtained in the lithotomy position after proper cleansing with the assistance of a nurse. Often urethral catheterization is necessary to obtain a clean specimen.

■ Infants

Suprapubic needle aspiration is usually the only effective method for obtaining a noncontaminated specimen for culture.

Gross Inspection

Color and appearance should be noted. A cloudy or milky appearance can be due to the precipitation of phosphates (phosphaturia) in alkaline urine, pyuria, or, rarely, chyluria.

Specific Gravity

Specific gravity, measured by hydrometer or refractometer, can give a good estimate of the patient's hydration, barring significant renal impairment. The normal range is 1.003 to 1.030. Glucose, protein, or intravenous contrast agents in the urine can cause a falsely elevated value.

Chemical Dipstick

The urine dipstick permits simultaneous performance of a battery of useful chemical tests in less than 2 minutes. These are screening tests, and positive results generally need confirmation by other more precise tests.

■ pH

pH is normally slightly acidic, except after a meal. A highly alkaline pH (>8) suggests infection with a urea-splitting organism such as *Proteus.*

■ Protein

Protein estimation by the dipstick can be a tip-off to significant disease such as glomerulopathy or cancer. Some other causes of positive protein readings include white cells, vaginal secretions, prolonged fever, and readings after excessive exercise. Persistently positive results must be confirmed by quantitative tests. Normal is less than 200 mg protein per 24-hour urine collection.

■ Glucose

Glucose determination by dipstick is both sensitive and specific, with most positive readings occurring in diabetics. False positives can result from large doses of aspirin, ascorbic acid (vitamin C), or cephalosporins.

■ Hemoglobin

Hemoglobin by dipstick is not specific for red cells; however, it is a good screening test. Positive results must be confirmed by microscopic analysis. Free hemoglobin and myoglobin will cause false-positive results. Ascorbic acid in the urine can cause false negatives. Dipsticks that have been left exposed to air will be inaccurate.

Microscopic Examination

Microscopy of the centrifuged urinary sediment is essential for every urinalysis.

▨ Procedure

Ten milliliters fresh urine is centrifuged at 2,000 rpm for 3 to 5 minutes. Nearly all supernatant is removed by turning the tube upside down. After returning to the upright position, the centrifuge tube is vigorously tapped to resuspend the sediment. This suspension is then tapped onto the glass slide and covered with a coverslip.

▨ Microscopy

Microscopy is first performed at low power [100× magnification (i.e., 10× objective)], looking specifically for cells, casts, trichomonads, or crystals. Once any of these elements is observed, then high power [400× magnification (i.e., 40× objective)] should be used for specific identification. The approximate volume of urine under a coverslip at high-power magnification is 1/20,000 to 1/50,000 of a milliliter.

Red Blood Cells

Red blood cells in the urine can be differentiated into two morphologic types: epithelial and glomerular.

Epithelial red blood cells are regular with smooth, rounded, or crenellated membranes and an even hemoglobin distribution. As few as one per high-power field (hpf) suggests urologic disease.

Glomerular red blood cells are dysmorphic with irregular shapes and cell membranes and minimal or uneven hemoglobin distribution. More than 1,000,000 are normally excreted in the urine over a 24-hour period. The upper limit of normal is 1,000/mL urine or one for every two hpf. Two or more per hpf suggest glomerulonephritis.

White Blood Cells

Generally more than five to eight white blood cells (WBCs)/hpf is considered abnormal (pyuria) in a properly collected specimen. This finding would justify empiric therapy in a patient with symptoms of infection. Clumping suggests a more severe inflammatory response. Causes of pyuria include urinary tract infection (pyelonephritis, cystitis, prostatitis, urethritis, etc.), renal tuberculosis (sterile pyuria), and urolithiasis.

Casts

Casts are formed in the distal tubules and collecting ducts from a mucoprotein matrix of the Tamm–Horsfall protein and cellular elements. They generally signify intrinsic renal disease.

Red blood cell casts are diagnostic of glomerular bleeding (i.e., glomerulonephritis).

White blood cell casts are rarely seen but suggest pyelonephritis. Peroxidase staining is necessary to confirm that they are indeed polymorphonuclear leukocytes.

Granular casts (coarse, fine, and waxy) represent sloughed renal tubular epithelial cells and indicate intrinsic renal tubular disease.

Squamous Epithelial Cells

Squamous epithelial cells in the sediment suggest contamination of the specimen (common in female patients).

Bacteria and Yeasts

As few as one bacterium per hpf in a strict, properly collected specimen indicates bacteriuria.

URINE CULTURE

The presumptive diagnosis of a urinary tract infection based on symptoms, and urinalysis should be confirmed by culture. Culture of a properly collected urine specimen (as described earlier) will provide identification, quantification, and specific antimicrobial sensitivities for the offending pathogen.

Bacterial Count

Infection is defined as 10^3 to 10^5 bacteria per milliliter in a properly collected specimen.

Technique for Urine Specimen Localization

Collecting the urine specimen in specific segmented samples is useful for localizing the source of a urinary tract infection or inflammatory process in male patients. Ensure that the patient has a full bladder and that the glans is properly prepared. Collect each specimen into a separate sterile container.

1. VB1—collect the first 10 mL voided (urethral sample)
2. VB2—collect a midstream sample after patient has voided about 200 mL (bladder sample)
3. Stop voiding
4. EPS— massage prostate and collect drops of prostate secretions (prostatic sample)
5. VB3—again have patient void immediately and collect first 10 mL (prostatic sample)

LABORATORY TESTS

Serum Creatinine

Serum creatinine is a simple measurement that accurately reflects the glomerular filtration rate (GFR). Creatinine is a metabolic product of creatine phosphate in skeletal muscle. The daily production is relatively stable for a given individual and is proportional to muscle mass. Creatinine clearance occurs mainly by glomerular filtration (90%) and, to a lesser extent, by tubular secretion (10%). Thus creatinine clearance approximates the GFR, and a doubling of serum creatinine indicates a 50% reduction in GFR. As individual nephrons (of the 1,000,000/kidney) are lost to disease, the remainder hypertrophy, and the single-nephron GFR increases to maintain the overall GFR. A loss of 40% to 50% of renal mass is required before the GFR begins to decrease and creatinine increases. Note: a normal creatinine in a term infant is only 0.1 to 0.4 mg/dL because of low muscle mass.

Blood Urea Nitrogen

Urea is a metabolic product of protein catabolism that is excreted by the kidneys. Blood levels tend to reflect the GFR but can be influenced by dietary protein intake, hydration, gastrointestinal bleeding, and glucocorticoids. The BUN/creatinine ratio, which is normally 10:1, can be a useful indicator.

■ Conditions with Elevated BUN/Creatinine Ratio

- Dehydration
- Prerenal azotemia
- Urinary tract obstruction
- Blood in gastrointestinal tract
- Increased tissue catabolism
- Increased dietary protein intake
- Treatment with glucocorticoids

Prostatic Acid Phosphatase

Acid phosphatase is an enzyme produced by various body tissues; however, the prostate is noted to be the most concentrated source. Human prostatic acid phosphatase (PAP) is a glycoprotein of 102,000 MW. Routine enzymatic serum assays specific for PAP use thymolphthalein phosphate as substrate. Blood samples should be chilled immediately after collection to avoid loss of enzyme activity. An elevated serum enzymatic PAP indicates metastatic disease. Routine enzymatic assays for PAP have 70% sensitivity and 90% specificity.

▩ Causes of False-Positive Serum Prostatic Acid Phosphatase

- Serum samples taken within 24 hours of prostatic massage or transurethral resection of the prostate
- Serum samples that contain red cell hemolysis
- Serum samples from patients with fever

Prostate-Specific Antigen

Prostate-specific antigen (PSA) is a 34-kDa glycoprotein found only in the cytoplasm of prostatic epithelial cells. It is believed to function as a neutral serine protease that lyses seminal coagulum. It can be detected in the semen and serum of men with prostate tissue. It cannot be detected in women. PSA is the most useful test for prostate cancer.

PSA is specific only for prostate tissue and cannot differentiate benign from malignant prostate conditions. However, serum PSA levels above the normal range of 0 to 4 ng/mL correlate well with the presence of prostate cancer. In addition to prostate cancer, serum PSA levels can be elevated by acute prostatitis, vigorous prostatic manipulation or surgery, and markedly enlarged benign prostate glands. Serum PSA has been used extensively in prostate cancer for early detection, staging, and monitoring response to therapy. Serum PSA screening has become the best means for detecting early prostate cancer. PSA levels greater than 10 ng/mL are highly suggestive of the presence of prostate cancer, even in men with a normal digital rectal examination. The level of serum PSA tends to correlate with age and the volume of prostate cancer.

The percentage of free PSA is a useful assay for differentiating a benign from malignant source of PSA when the PSA level is between 4.0 and 10.0 ng/mL. A low percentage of free PSA (<15%) increases the likelihood that prostate cancer is present.

Alkaline Phosphatase

Alkaline phosphatase is an enzyme produced by many tissues, especially bone, liver, intestine, and placenta. Most enzyme present in normal serum is derived from metabolic activity in bone. Prostate cancer metastatic to bone causes an elevation in alkaline phosphatase secondary to increased metabolic activity in the bone surrounding the metastatic lesion. When an elevated total alkaline phosphatase is in question, the bone-derived isoenzyme can be isolated by its heat lability (bone burns). If the enzymatic activity of the heated fraction is less than 30% of the total, it suggests bone as the origin (bone isoenzyme is inactivated by heating).

24-Hour Urine Collection

A 24-hour collection is often necessary for the workup of stone-forming patients and for an accurate assessment of renal function or proteinuria in a patient with renal disease. The most common reason for inaccuracy of values obtained from a 24-hour urine collection is incomplete collection. An incomplete collection is suggested by an inadequate amount of total creatinine in the sample because the total amount of creatinine excreted in 24 hours is dependent on muscle mass and is generally constant. The normal production of creatinine is 1.0 mg/kg per hour.

▓ Stone Workup

A 24-hour urine collection for calcium, phosphorus, oxalate, magnesium, citrate, and uric acid is standard in the evaluation of the repeated stone former.

▓ Creatinine Clearance

Creatinine clearance can be calculated from a 24-hour urine collection by knowing the volume of urine in milliliters per 24 hours (V), urine creatinine concentration in milligrams per milliliter (U_c), plasma creatinine concentration in milligrams per milliliter (P_c), and the following formula: (1,440 min/24 hr)

$$C_{creat}(mL/min) = \frac{U_{creat}(V/1,440)}{P_{creat}}$$

Creatinine clearance can be estimated without a 24-hour urine collection simply by knowing the patient's age, sex, weight, and serum creatinine and using the following formula.

$$C_{creat} = \frac{(140 - age)(weight\ in\ kg)}{}$$

Multiply answer by 0.85 for females.

This formula is invalid in the setting of acute renal failure because its application requires a stable serum creatinine (steady state).

▓ Proteinuria

Normal 24-hour protein excretion is less than 200 mg. Heavy proteinuria (>2 g/day) is suggestive of glomerular disease.

Urinary Electrolytes

Spot urinary sodium (Na) and potassium (K) measurements can be a valuable tool in diagnosing hypovolemia or prerenal azotemia. The kidney has an impressive capacity to hold onto sodium.

Human Chorionic Gonadotropin

Human chorionic gonadotropin (hCG) is a 38,000-MW double-chain glycoprotein with α- and β-subunits normally secreted by the syncytiotrophoblastic cells of the placenta. hCG is elevated in all patients with choriocarcinoma, in 40% to 60% of embryonal carcinomas, and in 5% to 10% of pure seminomas. Its α-subunit is similar to those of luteinizing hormone, follicle-stimulating hormone, and thyroid-stimulating hormone; therefore, antibodies to the β-subunit must be used for measurement. It has a metabolic half-life of 24 hours, and normal adult levels should be less than 5 mIU/mL (see Chapter 26).

α-Fetoprotein

α-Fetoprotein (AFP) is a 70,000-MW single-chain glycoprotein normally secreted by the fetal yolk sac. It also is produced by trophoblastic cells of embryonal carcinoma and yolk sac tumors. It is *not* made by pure choriocarcinoma or seminoma. Elevated AFP is found in 50% to 70% of nonseminomatous testis tumors. It has a half-life of 4 to 6 days, and normal adult levels should be less than 40 ng/mL (see Chapter 26).

IMAGING TECHNIQUES

Roentgen Rays and Radiation

X-rays are electromagnetic waves of energy created when high-speed electrons hit the tungsten target of an x-ray tube. They fluoresce and expose photographic film while having great penetrating ability. An x-ray is ionizing energy owing to its ability to liberate electrons from atoms. The radiation dose is measured in terms of the ionizing energy absorbed by the tissues, and its unit is the rad (radiation absorbed dose). One hundred rads is equal to one gray (100 rads = 1 Gy; 1 mGy = 0.1 rad). The rem or sievert (Sv) is a radiation unit that defines the biologic effect of the dose on tissues (1 Sv = 100 rem; 1 mSv = 0.1 rem); however, for x-rays, one rad or Gy equals one rem or Sv. Today Gy and Sv are the preferred units of measure. The average yearly background environmental exposure in the United States ranges from 80 to 125 mrem [1 mrem (millirem) = 10^{-3} rem] per person. In medical diagnostic radiographs, less than 1% of the ionizing radiation passes through the patient unimpeded, whereas 99% is absorbed. According to the National Council on Radiation Protection and Measurements, the recommended permissible annual occupational radiation exposure limit is 50 mGy/year whole-body dose.

■ Radiation Exposure Hazard

- A linear relationship exists between dose and carcinogenicity for doses of more than 1 Gy.
- A whole-body dose of 5 Gy can be fatal.
- Radiation dose is cumulative over a person's lifetime.
- Scatter radiation is the principal source of hazard to x-ray personnel and urologists using fluoroscopy.
- A chest radiograph has an effective dose of 0.02 mSv (1 mSv = 1 mGy for radiographs).
- An IVU is equivalent to 125 chest radiographs or close to 1 year of natural background radiation.
- An abdominal CT scan is equivalent to 500 chest radiographs or 3.3 years of natural background radiation.
- Eye exposure causes cataracts.

■ How to Avoid Scatter Radiation Exposure

- Use lead aprons, thyroid shields, and lead eyeglasses when in the same room as the active x-ray source.
- Maximize your distance from the x-ray source (remember the inverse-square law: exposure rate decreases with square of the distance).
- Minimize fluoroscopic times.
- Use fluoroscopic machines only with the x-ray tube under the table.

Contrast Media

Use of iodinated contrast media greatly enhances radiographic studies of the urinary tract. Sodium or methylglucamine salts of triiodinated benzoic acid (Renografin; Hypaque), referred to as high-osmolality contrast media (HOCM), were the most frequently used contrast media for intravenous urography (IVU). Routine dosages are 1 mL/kg or 0.5 mL/lb of standard-strength urographic contrast agents given by rapid IV push. The mortality rate associated with the administration of contrast agents is approximately 1 per 50,000 patients. Use of nonionic low-osmolality contrast media (LOCM) such as iohexol (Omnipaque), iopamidol (Isovue), or ioversol (Optiray) has been shown to decrease adverse effects markedly.

■ Adverse Effects of Iodinated Contrast Media

Vasomotor Effects

Vasomotor effects, including a sensation of warmth or flushing, nausea, vomiting, or a metallic taste, occur in up to 50% of patients and are of no clinical significance.

Anaphylactoid Reactions

Allergic reactions usually occur immediately or within 5 to 10 minutes and are characterized by hypotension and tachycardia when severe. Mild to moderate erythema and urticaria occur in up to 5% of patients and can be treated with 50 mg diphenhydramine (Benadryl) IM, if necessary. Severe urticaria or any respiratory distress, including burning or tightness of the throat, change in voice, laryngeal edema, bronchospasm, or apnea, occurs in up to 1 in 1,000 patients and should be treated with immediate epinephrine (1:1,000) 0.3 to 0.5 mg SC, followed by the usual resuscitation efforts, as needed.

Vagal Reactions

Vagal reactions are characterized by hypotension and bradycardia when severe. Early signs are confusion, apprehension, and diaphoresis. Severe bradycardia (heart rate <50 beats/min) and hypotension (systolic blood pressure <80 mm Hg) should be treated with intravenous fluids, leg elevation, and 0.5 to 1.0 mg atropine IV push to increase heart rate.

Nephrotoxicity

Nephrotoxicity is believed to be dose related and is therefore dependent on extracellular fluid volume and renal function. It usually manifests as a decrease in urine output and a modest increase in serum creatinine within 24 hours, which peaks 2 to 5 days after the procedure. Patients with type I insulin-dependent diabetes and a serum creatinine of greater than 1.5 have been noted to be at high risk of nephrotoxicity. Diabetics taking Glucophage should discontinue medication for 48 hours after IV contrast is used. Patients with normal renal function (creatinine <1.5), even if diabetic, generally have a negligible risk of nephrotoxicity as long as large doses of contrast are avoided. An advantage for LOCM over HOCM in nephrotoxicity is unclear.

Cardiovascular Toxicity

Hypertonicity and direct chemotoxic effects can result in intravascular volume expansion, hemodilution, and hypotension in patients with cardiac risk factors.

▓ Risk Factors for Adverse Effects from Contrast Media

- Diabetes (type I, juvenile) with renal insufficiency (creatinine >1.5 mg/dL)
- Renal insufficiency (creatinine >1.5 mg/dL)
- Diabetics taking metformin (Glucophage)
- Dehydration
- History of a previous reaction to contrast media
- History of allergic diseases [e.g., hayfever, asthma, food (especially shellfish) allergies]
- Congestive heart failure (effective volume depletion)
- Multiple myeloma

▓ Prevention of Adverse Effects of Contrast Media

- Identify high-risk patients.
- Keep patient well hydrated (avoid use of strong laxatives).
- Premedicate with steroids (hydrocortisone 100 mg PO or prednisone 20 mg PO q6h × 3 doses before study and diphenhydramine 50 mg PO) those patients who are at increased risk of an allergic-like reaction.
- Use nonionic contrast agents (Omnipaque).
- Hold Glucophage for 48 hours after contrast administration.

Ultrasound

Ultrasound is an extremely desirable method of imaging many urologic structures in a quick, cost-efficient, and noninvasive manner, without radiation or other known hazards. The advent of high-frequency, gray-scale, B-mode real-time scanning has greatly improved ultrasound images; however, they remain somewhat operator dependent. Bone and air are poor conductors of sound and thus block images of structures behind them. Fat also limits conduction; thus obese patients are difficult to image. Water conducts well and appears sonolucent. Sound is reflected whenever it encounters an interface of different tissue densities. Color-flow

Doppler ultrasound can give valuable information regarding the perfusion and vascularity of the organ.

▦ Renal Ultrasound

Renal ultrasound is especially useful when evaluating the kidney for cysts, solid masses, abscesses, hydronephrosis, stones, perirenal masses, and transplant rejection. The right kidney can be imaged with the patient supine, by using the liver as an acoustic window, or posteriorly. The left kidney is generally viewed posteriorly or with the patient in a right lateral decubitus position by using the spleen as an acoustic window.

Criteria for a Simple Benign Cyst
- No echoes within mass
- Good through transmission—acoustic enhancement distal to lesion
- Sharply marginated, smooth posterior wall

Criteria for Transplant Rejection
- Enlargement from edema
- Indistinct corticomedullary junction
- Loss of central renal-sinus fat echo

Indications for Renal Ultrasound
- Differentiate a cystic from solid mass (95% accurate)
- Evaluate for obstruction (98% sensitivity and 90% specificity in detecting hydronephrosis)
- Evaluate renal transplants for evidence of rejection or obstruction
- Look for stones

▦ Bladder Ultrasound

Bladder ultrasound can be performed transabdominally, transurethrally, or transrectally. It is used to assess bladder filling and to estimate postvoid residual urine.

▦ Prostate Ultrasound—Transrectal Ultrasound of Prostate

Transrectal ultrasound of the prostate (TRUSP) cannot differentiate benign from malignant prostate tissue. It is not a screening test for detection of prostate cancer. The primary reasons to use TRUSP are to guide prostate needle biopsies and to measure the size of the prostate (see Chapter 22).

▦ Scrotal Ultrasound

Scrotal ultrasound is most valuable in differentiating intratesticular from extratesticular processes with an accuracy of 90% to

100%. This is important because most intratesticular lesions are solid and malignant, and most extratesticular lesions are cystic and benign. It is also of some help in detecting testicular rupture when suspicion is low. Color-flow Doppler ultrasound can differentiate testicular torsion from epididymitis (see Chapter 10).

Radiographs

■ Chest Radiograph
Chest radiographs should be a part of every metastatic workup.

■ Plain Film
Plain film [also referred to as flat plate, scout film, or kidney, ureter, and bladder (KUB)] is an invaluable aid in diagnosis and should not be underestimated. Pay careful attention to the size and shape of the renal outlines, and look for the presence of calcifications or air patterns.

Calcifications on Plain Film
- Urinary calculi—90% are opaque (70%–90% of ureteral calculi can be found on KUB)
- Parenchymal calcifications within cysts or tumors (calcification increases likelihood of malignancy)
- Nephrocalcinosis (hyperparathyroidism, renal tubular acidosis, medullary sponge kidney)
- Tuberculosis of kidney
- Adrenal calcifications (suggests a history of adrenal hemorrhage)
- Phleboliths
- Calcified lymph nodes
- Gallstones (10% are calcified)
- Appendicolith (fecalith—helpful if acute appendicitis is suspected)
- Calcified costal cartilages
- Calcified uterine fibroids
- Prostatic calcifications (suggests chronic prostatitis)
- Aortic calcifications
- Pancreatic calcification (suggests pancreatitis)

Air under Diaphragm
- Ruptured hollow viscus (emergency)
- Postoperative

Air within Kidney or Renal Pelvis

- Emphysematous pyelonephritis

Enlargement of One Kidney	Enlargement of Both Kidneys
Renal tumor or cyst	Polycystic kidney disease
Unilateral hydronephrosis	Bilateral hydronephrosis
Unilateral acute renal vein thrombosis	Amyloidosis, multiple myeloma, etc.
Compensatory hypertrophy	Glycogen storage diseases
Multicystic kidney disease	

Unilateral Small Kidney	Bilateral Small Kidneys
Congenital hypoplastic kidney	End-stage renal disease
Chronic pyelonephritis with scarring	Arteriosclerosis, nephrosclerosis
	Chronic glomerulonephritis
Renal artery stenosis	Papillary necrosis

Intravenous Urography

Intravenous urography (IVU, IVP) remains one of the best diagnostic methods for obtaining anatomic and functional detail of the urinary tract. Routinely, 50 to 100 mL of contrast media is rapidly injected by IV push, followed by 1-, 5-, 10-, and 20-minute films, which are carefully monitored by a radiologist, and a postvoid film. The IVU is the gold standard for evaluating the patient with hematuria, and it is more sensitive than ultrasound in diagnosing acute hydronephrosis and in detecting ureteral or renal calculi.

■ Tomograms

Tomograms of the kidney during IVU are essential to obtain maximal detail of renal anatomy and are usually performed after the 1-minute film of a standard IVU.

Retrograde Urography

Retrograde urography can be performed only during cystoscopy. It is an extremely valuable procedure, when indicated, because it gives excellent definition of upper-tract anatomy. Technique will vary depending on whether a pyelogram or ureterogram is of primary interest. Generally an opaque whistle-tip or open-ended ureteral catheter can be passed up the ureter, or a bulb or acorn-tipped catheter can be placed in the ureteral orifice, followed by injection of 4 to 8 mL of half-strength Renografin into the catheter. Care must be taken to eliminate air bubbles. Appropriate films are taken, followed by a drainage film 10 minutes after removing the catheter. Antibiotic coverage should be used. Complications include ureteral perforation, pyelonephritis, ureteral edema, and contrast absorption in the upper tract with systemic reaction.

■ Indications for Retrograde Pyelography

- Poor renal function
- Poor visualization on IVU
- Equivocal findings on IVU
- Patients at high risk for contrast reactions
- Localizing level of ureteral obstruction

Anterograde Urography

Percutaneous studies are valuable when excretory or retrograde studies are contraindicated, particularly in infants and children, or when a nephrostomy tube is already in place. The contrast agent is directly injected into the collecting system via a percutaneous puncture through the patient's flank. Antibiotic coverage should be used. Contraindications include a bleeding diathesis, a nondilated collecting system, or local skin infection.

Retrograde Urethrogram

Retrograde urethrogram is used to demonstrate the anterior urethra (penile, bulbar, and membranous portions). A 12 F Foley catheter is placed into the urethra just until the base of the balloon disappears through the meatus. The balloon is then filled with 1 to 2 mL water, just enough to keep the catheter within the fossa navicularis with gentle resistance. Films are taken in the right posterior oblique position while injecting 30 to 50 mL half-strength standard contrast media.

Voiding Cystourethrogram

Voiding cystourethrogram (VCUG) is used to demonstrate the posterior urethra (bladder neck and prostatic urethra) or for demonstration of vesicoureteral reflux. It also is valuable in demonstrating the bladder and bladder-neck function in women with incontinence. The bladder is first filled, after urethral catheterization or suprapubic puncture. Dilute (15%) standard contrast medium is dripped by gravity from 45 cm above the level of the bladder until a sensation of discomfort is experienced. Films are taken in the right or left posterior oblique position while the patient voids. A VCUG also can be performed when the bladder is full after an excretory urogram (however, reflux cannot be assessed in this setting).

■ Indications for Voiding Cystourethrogram

- Urinary tract infections in children and recurrent or persistent infections in adults
- Suspicion of vesicoureteral reflux
- Suspicion of posterior urethral valves
- Posterior urethral strictures
- Hydronephrosis in children
- Neurogenic bladders
- Urinary incontinence (cystocele, residual urine)

Computed Tomography

Computed tomography (CT) scans use computer-generated images of cross-sectional anatomy by interpretation of x-ray–derived attenuation values through finite portions of a body slice. The CT picture is composed of tiny picture elements (pixels) to which 16 shades of gray are assigned. Each pixel actually represents a volume element (voxel) of tissue within a slice. Voxels are represented by an arbitrary scale of CT numbers or Hounsfield units (HU) from –1,000 to +1,000, with 0 HU equal to water. Because only 16 pixel shades are available to represent 2,000 HU, many voxels will appear the same shade of gray in the CT picture. Soft-tissue definition in body CT scans is routinely improved by limiting the range of HUs represented to 400 (–200 to +200). This is performed by setting the window width to 400 HU while maintaining a center of 0 HU. Use of both oral and intravenous contrast agents enhances CT images. New helical (spiral) CT scanners are faster and more accurate and minimize partial-volume artifacts seen in axial scanning.

■ Relative Hounsfield Units for Various Tissues	
Air	–1,000 HU
Fat	–150 to –50 HU
Water, bile, cerebrospinal fluid	0 (±20)
Soft tissues	30–70 HU
Fresh blood, calcium	80 HU
Dense cortical bone	+1,000 HU

▨ Common Problems in Interpreting Computed Tomography Scans

1. Hounsfield units can be unreliable.
   a. Variable calibration standards
   b. Partial-volume effect
   c. Patient-motion artifacts
   d. Streak artifacts (bone, barium, metal clips, air–fluid levels)
   e. Computer-generated artifacts
2. Intestinal lumen must be opacified with contrast.
3. CT has limited value in identifying lymph node metastases (especially in transitional cell carcinoma and prostate cancer) because of poor sensitivity (60%–70%).
4. CT cannot distinguish postoperative, postradiation, or postchemotherapy fibrosis from residual tumor.
5. Very obese or very thin, emaciated patients do not scan well.
6. Window width and center should be noted if the image is unusual.
7. Anatomic variants may be present.
   a. Gastric fundus posterior to pancreas
   b. Prominent medial lobe of spleen
   c. Accessory spleens
   d. Renal lobulation
   e. Left-sided or duplicated IVC
8. CT cannot differentiate among an infected cyst, hemorrhagic cyst, abscess, area of infarction or tumor necrosis, and metastases.

▨ Computed Tomography Criteria for a Benign Simple Renal Cyst

- Smooth, thin, invisible wall
- Homogeneous water density (0 HU ±20)
- No contrast enhancement
- Sharp margination and interface with adjacent renal parenchyma

▨ Specific Computed Tomography Scan Protocols

1. *Stone protocol*—helical (spiral) CT scanning of the abdomen and pelvis is performed without oral or N contrast for acute evaluation of colic for a suspected stone. Its advantage is speed, no need for contrast, and even radiolucent uric acid stones will be seen. If no stone or hydronephrosis is found, a stone can reliably be ruled out. However, it often fails to define the degree of obstruction. A follow-up IVU may be necessary.
2. *Renal protocol*—CT scanning to evaluate a renal mass must be performed first without and then with IV contrast. Hypodense lesions on noncontrast scans that enhance with IV contrast are solid and considered renal cell carcinoma until proven

otherwise. Fat within a solid renal mass is strong presumptive evidence for an angiomyolipoma.

Angiograms

Renal arteriography allows excellent anatomic visualization of the renal anatomy. In brief, the technique first involves placement of a catheter into the femoral artery by using the Seldinger method followed by an initial bolus aortogram. Next, selective renal arteriography may be performed for detail of the intrarenal vascular bed. The patient commonly receives 50 to 75 mL contrast agent during the entire procedure. Indications for renal arteriography have diminished considerably in recent years because of the remarkable advances in ultrasound, CT scans, and magnetic resonance imaging (MRI).

■ Complications of Renal Arteriography

1. Contrast-related injury
   a. Allergic reactions
   b. Nephrotoxicity (acute tubular necrosis)
2. Procedure-related injury
   a. Local bleeding, hematoma
   b. Arterial thrombosis
   c. Arterial dissection
   d. Thromboembolization to lower extremity
   e. False aneurysm formation
   f. Arteriovenous fistulae

■ Indications for Renal Arteriography

1. Preoperative for renal vascular anatomy
2. Renal trauma (when indicated)
3. Living-donor renal transplants [digital subtraction angiography (DSA) generally preferred]
4. Workup of renovascular hypertension (DSA preferred)
5. Suspicion of renal artery aneurysm
6. Renal tumors (before partial nephrectomy)
7. Renal artery embolization

Digital Subtraction Angiography

DSA combines x-rays, contrast media, and digital computer technology to produce a high-quality angiographic image with certain technical advantages. In brief, a mask image is first made of the area of interest, before contrast enhancement, and it is digitally stored in memory. After contrast enhancement, multiple subtraction images are made of the identical area and stored in memory. The enhanced images can then be subtracted from the original mask image, leaving only the contrast-enhanced structures (i.e., vascular anatomy) with no background. The only major problem with DSA is that any patient motion will degrade the images because precise registration between the mask and subtraction images is necessary.

■ Two Types of Digital Subtraction Angiography

1. Intravenous DSA (IV-DSA) is performed by peripheral or central venous injection of 40 to 50 mL contrast agent, usually central, followed by routine DSA. It is the procedure of choice in the initial evaluation of suspected renovascular hypertension and for evaluation of renal transplant donors. Advantages of IV-DSA are (a) it avoids the significant risks of arterial catheterization and (b) it is an outpatient procedure that does not require the expense of hospitalization.
2. Intraarterial DSA (IA-DSA) uses arterial catheterization with DSA technology. Its chief advantage is that only minimal amounts of contrast agent are needed (<10 mL), making it particularly useful in patients with renal failure.

Venography

■ Renal Venography

Renal venography is helpful in detecting renal vein thrombosis with either clot or tumor thrombus. Renal vein catheterization also is used for measuring renal vein renin activity in patients with suspected renovascular hypertension.

■ Venacavography

Venacavography is often a useful adjunct to CT or MRI in defining the extent of involvement of the vena cava with renal tumor thrombus.

Lymphangiograms

Lymphangiograms are performed by direct catheterization of a lymphatic vessel on the dorsum of the foot with a fine (27- or 30-gauge) needle and injecting contrast media (Ethiodol). Lymphangiograms were more commonly used in the past to aid diagnosis of lymph node metastases in prostate, bladder, and testicular malignancies. However, because of their poor sensitivity in detecting lymph node involvement in pelvic (50%) and retroperitoneal (75%) locations, they are no longer routinely used. Indications for pedal lymphangiography include the following:

- Patients with stage I testicular germ cell tumors who are candidates for surveillance;
- Planning of radiotherapy portals.

Nuclear Scans

Nuclear scans use radioactive tracers, primarily technetium-99m (^{99m}Tc) chelates and iodine-131 (^{131}I) orthoiodohippurate, to derive functional images and data by using the Anger scintillation camera.

■ DMSA Renal Scan

^{99m}Tc-DMSA is not filtered but binds to the basement membrane of proximal tubular cells ($t_{1/2}$, 6 hr). It is used to assess functional renal mass and differential or relative renal function between the two kidneys. Optimal scanning is performed 4 or 24 hours after injection of tracer.

Indications for DMSA Renal Scan

- Estimation of differential renal function
- Estimation of functioning renal mass
- Evaluation of a pseudotumor
- Assessment of pyelonephritis in children

■ DTPA Renal Scan (with or without Lasix)

^{99m}Tc-DTPA is excreted principally in the urine by glomerular filtration (80%) and is not secreted or reabsorbed ($t_{1/2}$, 1.4 hr). It is used to assess renal blood flow, GFR, and the functional status of the collecting systems (i.e., obstruction). Patients must be well hydrated.

The renogram produced is a time–activity curve of renal function consisting of three phases:

1. *Vascular phase*—represents primarily renal perfusion (normally a steep upward curve lasting <1 min);
2. *Tubular-uptake phase*—represents the gradual accumulation of activity in the parenchyma [transit time (i.e., time to peak activity) is normally 3–5 min];
3. *Excretory phase*—represents washout of activity that depends on rate of urine production and flow in the collecting system (normally a steep downward sloping curve with a washout $t_{1/2}$

of 10 minutes). By administering furosemide (Lasix) during the washout phase, a dilated, nonobstructed system can usually be differentiated from a truly obstructed system.

Indications for DTPA Renogram

- Evaluation of renal transplant function
- Diagnosis of upper-tract obstruction
- Evaluation of a renal mass in the newborn

▨ MAG3 Renal Scan (with or without Lasix)

^{99m}Tc-MAG3 is handled by almost exclusively (90%) tubular secretion. It is believed to be superior to DTPA for diuretic renography to determine the presence or absence of obstruction in the hydronephrotic kidney.

Indications for MAG3 Renogram

- To determine the presence or absence of obstruction in the hydronephrotic kidney
- To evaluate ureteropelvic junction obstruction

▨ Hippuran Scan

^{131}I-Hippuran (orthoiodohippurate) is excreted in the urine by tubular secretion (80%) and glomerular filtration (20%). It measures effective renal plasma flow, a more accurate indicator of excretory function. ^{131}I-Hippuran should be used when looking for obstruction in the presence of significant renal failure, because glomerular function is affected earlier and to a greater extent than tubular function.

▨ Radionuclide Cystography

Radionuclide cystography is effective for evaluation of vesicoureteral reflux in the pediatric patient. It is more sensitive than a VCUG and gives 50 to 200 times less radiation exposure. It is performed either by direct retrograde filling of the bladder with ^{99m}Tc-pertechnetate in saline or indirectly after a routine DTPA renal scan (less accurate).

▨ Testicular Flow Scan

Testicular flow scan using ^{99m}Tc-pertechnetate for the differentiation of testicular torsion from epididymitis has a reported 95% sensitivity and 100% specificity.

Common Patterns

- Acute early torsion—decreased perfusion to the involved side
- Late or missed torsion—central photon deficiency with a halo or rim of reactive hyperemia on delayed images

- Epididymitis—increased perfusion to the involved side and a crescent of increased activity corresponding to the inflamed epididymitis

Bone Scan

A bone scan is the most sensitive means of detecting osseous metastases (≤97%). Positive bone scans often precede radiographic lesions by 3 to 6 months. ^{99m}Tc-Methylene-diphosphonate, the most useful agent, is taken up in all areas of increased bone turnover, not just metastatic deposits. However, metastatic lesions characteristically are asymmetrical, multiple, and involve the axial skeleton. False negatives occur in 3% to 8% of cases. Normally, the kidneys are seen to take up isotope. Failure to visualize the kidneys indicates either inadequate tracer dose or that widespread metastatic disease has taken up all the isotope (superscan). Serial scans are often misleading in evaluating response to hormonal therapy or chemotherapy.

Indications for Bone Scan

- Initial evaluation of prostate cancer and neuroblastoma
- Skeletal pain or other evidence of metastases in prostate cancer, renal cell cancer, seminoma, neuroblastoma, and bladder cancer (rarely)

Gallium Scan

Gallium-67 citrate scans are useful in patients with a suspected abscess and a nondiagnostic ultrasound. Imaging must wait 48 to 72 hours after injection because of normal urinary excretion. It is reported to have a sensitivity of 90%, but a specificity of only 65%, meaning that many false-positive scans occur.

Indium-111 Leukocyte Scan

Indium-111 oxine–labeled white blood cells require laboratory labeling of white cells; however, it is more sensitive and specific for localizing acute infections, and images can be made in less than 24 hours.

Positron Emission Tomography (PET) Scans

PET scans use a radioactive tracer, fluorodeoxyglucose (FDG). The scan tracks the uptake and utilization of FDG by cells about an hour after injection. It can be used to differentiate normal cells from malignant cells. PET scans have had limited use for urologic malignancies to date.

Magnetic Resonance Imaging

MRI gives outstanding soft-tissue resolution that is well suited for renal and adrenal masses and vascular imaging. Radiofrequency pulses are used to excite briefly the hydrogen protons of the tissues and organs to be imaged. Nuclear magnetic resonance (NMR) signals are characterized by (a) spin density, (b) T_1 relaxation time, and (c) T_2 relaxation time. A computer transforms NMR signals into a visual image by using a gray scale that corresponds to the signal intensity. Fat gives off the highest-intensity signal and is represented by white, whereas bone and air give the lowest signals and are represented by black. MRI can be enhanced by use of an intravascular contrast agent such as gadolinium-DTPA. T_1-weighted images are best for defining anatomy, whereas T_2-weighted images are better for demonstrating pathology. Cysts appear much brighter than solid masses on T_2-weighted images.

■ Indications for MRI

- Characterization of renal masses as solid or cystic.
- Imaging adrenal masses; presence of fat favors adenoma rather than metastasis.
- Pheochromocytomas are extremely bright on T_2-weighted images.
- MR angiography of kidneys (renal vein and vena cava patency).

■ Contraindications to MRI

- Pacemakers
- Ferromagnetic intracranial aneurysm clips
- Claustrophobia

ENDOSCOPY

The ability to visualize directly almost the entire urinary tract is one highlight of the specialty of urology. Modern fiberoptic light sources and wide-angle lenses provide a capability for precise diagnosis and follow-up that is unmatched by any specialty [note: French (F) scale; 3 F = 1 mm].

Urethroscopy

Urethroscopy is performed by using 0- or 30-degree lenses. Cystoscope sheaths range from 8 F to 26 F in caliber. Inspection for tumors, strictures, stones, diverticula, prostatic enlargement, and so on is conducted. A flexible cystoscope is preferred for an awake male patient.

■ Cystoscopy

Cystoscopy is possible by passing the scope into the bladder. Complete visualization of the entire bladder can generally be performed with 30- and 70-degree lenses. Inspection of the ureteral orifices and bladder walls for tumors, diverticula, lesions, stones, foreign bodies, and general morphology (i.e., trabeculation) can be conducted. A flexible cystoscope is preferred for an awake male patient.

Ureteroscopy

Transurethral ureteroscopy can be performed with rigid or flexible ureteroscopes, allowing visualization of the entire ureter up into the renal pelvis and major calyces.

Nephroscopy

Nephroscopy can be performed percutaneously with a rigid or flexible instrument. Many procedures are possible through the instrument. A small-caliber flexible ureteroscope can be passed into the renal pelvis for visualization of the intrarenal collecting system.

CYST PUNCTURE

Although most renal cysts are benign, and more than 90% can be correctly diagnosed with ultrasound or CT, some will require a cyst puncture to make a final diagnosis.

Technique

Cyst puncture is performed with a thin needle guided by ultrasound or CT. Cyst fluid is aspirated and sent for histochemical and cytologic studies followed by double-contrast (air-contrast media) imaging of the cyst cavity, taking multiple radiographic views.

Interpretation

■ Benign Cysts

Benign cysts contain a clear, straw-colored fluid with low levels of fat and protein, no blood, and negative cytology.

■ Malignant Cysts

Malignant cysts often have a murky or bloody fluid, with high concentrations of fat and protein, and positive cytology. Tumor nodules may be seen on the cyst walls.

■ Inflammatory Cysts

Inflammatory cysts have a murky or purulent aspirate with moderately elevated fat and protein concentrations and significant levels of amylase and lactate dehydrogenase. Cytology will show numerous inflammatory cells, and cultures will generally be positive.

PROSTATIC NEEDLE BIOPSY

Prostatic needle biopsy is essential for the diagnosis of prostate cancer. It is an easy, efficient, outpatient procedure that should be performed without hesitation for any suggestive areas found on digital rectal examination or with an elevated PSA (see Chapters 3 and 22). Ultrasound guidance should always be used if available. Two techniques are used: core-needle biopsy and fine-needle aspiration.

Core-Needle Biopsy

Core-needle biopsy is performed by using a spring-loaded Biopty needle via a transperineal or transrectal approach. Core biopsies yield good tissue samples for pathologic examination.

■ Transrectal

Transrectal ultrasound guided-needle biopsy is the standard for prostate biopsy. It allows accurate needle guidance and does not require an anesthetic. Six to 12 systematic random biopsies are taken under ultrasound guidance. Patients should hold aspirin and any anticoagulant or antiplatelet medications for approximately 5 to 7 days before biopsy. All patients should have a Fleets enema before biopsy and should have antibiotic coverage before and for 2 to 5 days after (generally a quinolone). Injection of lidocaine (Xylocaine) with a long needle into the periprostatic soft tissues at the prostate–vesical junction will greatly eliminate most of the discomfort of the procedure. Complications include bleeding, infection, urosepsis, and urinary retention.

■ **Transperineal**

Transperineal approach is less frequently used today. It does not conform with transrectal ultrasound as well and requires local anesthesia to the perineum. After local lidocaine (Xylocaine) infiltration of the perineum, the index finger of one hand is placed in the rectum to guide the needle held in the other hand toward the area in question.

Fine-Needle Aspiration

Aspiration by using a Franzen needle and transrectal approach has the lowest complication rate. Cells are aspirated through a thin 22-gauge needle for cytologic examination. It is performed as an outpatient procedure without anesthesia, and results can be available within hours.

CYTOLOGY

Cytology has expanded the capabilities of making early diagnosis from minimally invasive procedures. Cytologic examination can be performed on aspirates from the prostate, kidney, and lymph nodes; washings from the bladder, ureter, and renal pelvis; and voided urines. Well-preserved cells are essential for accurate interpretation. Difficulty most often arises in differentiating atypia from low-grade tumors.

FLOW CYTOMETRY

Flow cytometry utilizes a highly complex machine that can measure frequency, size, structure, and staining characteristics of thousands of cells per second. Studies have demonstrated significant associations between cell DNA ploidy and disease prognosis.

THE WHITAKER TEST

The Whitaker test is a quantitative pressure flow study used to evaluate upper-tract obstruction as from a ureteropelvic junction obstruction or an obstructed megaureter. It is considered the definitive test for obstruction when other less invasive methods are equivocal.

Procedure for a Whitaker Test

1. A nephrostomy or pyelostomy tube is placed in the renal pelvis (percutaneous 20-gauge needle nephrostomy is commonly used), and a catheter is placed in the bladder.
2. A constant-flow infusion is delivered to the renal pelvis at 10 mL/min.
3. Manometers are attached to perfusion and bladder outflow catheters.
4. Renal pelvis and bladder pressures are monitored once the collecting system is full.
5. Differential pressures (renal pelvis minus bladder) of less than 15 cm H_2O indicate absence of obstruction.

URODYNAMICS

Urodynamics is the study of physiology and fluid mechanics of normal and abnormal micturition. It encompasses a large field of specialized tests and nomenclature. Elaborate urodynamic studies require special equipment and training for proper performance. The two most useful and commonly used urodynamic studies are the uroflow and cystometrogram (see also Chapter 21).

Uroflow

The urine flow rate is ideally obtained on an electronic uroflowmeter that produces a flow curve that plots the instantaneous stream flow rate against time, in addition to measuring peak and average flow rates, flow time, and volume voided (see Chapter 21). Uroflow is the single most valuable urodynamic study to evaluate voiding dysfunction. The peak flow rate and the flow curve can confirm a diagnostic suspicion and provide etiologic insight into the voiding problem.

Cystometrogram

The cystometrogram is a recording of detrusor function using either a gas (CO_2) or water cystometer. Intravesical pressures are recorded during passive filling and active contraction of the bladder. Subjective events (first desire to void, sensation of fullness, and discomfort) are noted on the graph. Bladder compliance can be calculated from the filling phase of the study ($\Delta V/\Delta P$).

▨ Normal Cystometrogram

See Chapter 21.

- Good accommodation during filling with pressures in the range of 10 cm H_2O
- No uninhibited contractions (involuntary pressure spikes of >15 cm H_2O)
- First desire to void at 100 to 200 mL
- Fullness at 300 to 400 mL
- Discomfort between 400 and 500 mL
- Good detrusor contraction with pressures reaching 30 cm H_2O in the female and 30 to 50 cm H_2O in the male patient

▨ Sources of Error in Routine Cystometrogram

- Inability to differentiate detrusor pressure elevations from intraabdominal pressure
- Too fast a filling rate
- Urethral catheter irritation
- CO_2 can irritate the bladder mucosa
- Patient misunderstanding instructions
- Movement artifacts

Suggested Readings

MAJOR UROLOGIC TEXTBOOKS

Belman AB, King LR, Kramer SA, eds. *Clinical pediatric urology*, 4th ed. London: Martin Dunitz, 2002.

Gillenwater JY, Grayhack JT, Howards SS, Mitchell ME, eds. *Adult and pediatric urology*, 4th ed. Philadelphia: Lippincott Williams & Wilkins, 2001.

Walsh PC, Retik AB, Vaughan ED, Wein AJ, eds. *Campbell's urology*, 8th ed. Philadelphia: WB Saunders, 2002.

SPECIALIZED TEXTBOOKS

Graham SD, Keane TE, Glenn JF, eds. *Glenn's urologic surgery*. Philadelphia: Lippincott Williams & Wilkins, 2004.

Hinman F, ed. *Atlas of pediatric urologic surgery*. Philadelphia: WB Saunders, 1994.

Hinman F, ed. *Atlas of urologic surgery*, 2nd ed. Philadelphia: WB Saunders, 1998.

Taneja SS, Smith RB, Ehrlich RM, eds. *Complications of urologic surgery*, 3rd ed. Philadelphia: WB Saunders, 2001.

Weiss MA, Mills SE. *Atlas of genitourinary tract disorders*. Philadelphia: Lippincott Williams & Wilkins, 1988.

PERIODICALS

Journal of Urology
Official journal of the American Urological Association
http://www.jurology.com or http://www.auanet.org
Urology
Official Publication of the Societe Internationale d' Urologie
http://www.us.elsevierhealth.com
AUA Update Series
http://www.auanet.org

BJU International
http://www.bjui.org/
Urologic Clinics of North America
http://www.us.elsevierhealth.com

INDEX

Note: Page numbers in *italics* indicate figures, and page numbers followed by "t" indicate tables concerning the subject.